HOLDING
ON TO
HOPE

**Finding the 'New You' after
a Traumatic Brain Injury**

NICOLE YEATES

Holding On To Hope:
Finding the 'New You' After a Traumatic Brain Injury
© Copyright 2020 **Nicole Yeates**

ISBN: 978-0-6489949-0-9

For more information, email

nicole@holdingontohope.com.au

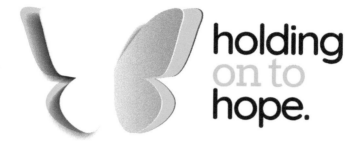

holding
on to
hope.

Tired of forgetting things and want to improve
your memory?

Why wait another day to improve?

GET YOUR FREE GIFT!

Free Memory Cheat Sheet & Retiink Memory
Management App Trial

Go the the following page to receive your free gift

https://www.holdingontohope.com.au/memory-
cheat-sheet

Dedication

I dedicate this book to all the friends and family who provided stimulation and support to me while I was in a coma, those who cared for me during my hospital stay, and those who stayed by my side through the most difficult rehabilitation pathway after release from hospital and beyond. The reality of my acquired disability was not fully realised until I returned home. Thank you to my family and friends who accepted the 'new me', without hesitation and despite the challenges.

The one constant, from beginning to end, has been my amazing and resilient mother, who has role modelled the most valuable personal attributes throughout my life. She continues to be an inspiration through her ability to power through seemingly insurmountable obstacles! Mum, you were the reason I did not want to leave this earth, and you have kept me on this earth many times over! I love you!

Table of Contents

Introduction

This book is written with a solution-focused framework specifically for people who have suffered a brain injury and for their carers or support persons. I have based it on my lived experience with traumatic brain injury (TBI) and 33 years of trial and error that have helped me navigate towards a productive and fulfilling life. Throughout this book, you will discover strategies for managing many of the barriers commonly associated with a TBI or acquired brain injury (ABI), such as short-term memory and concentration issues, fatigue, isolation, and coping with a negative prognosis.

If you are the carer or support person for someone with a brain injury, this book will also provide you with strategies to proactively assist the brain-injured person during the acute and non-acute phases and to advocate within health care systems, while also taking care of you.

A severe brain injury at age 16 transformed my life forever. My medical team did not expect me to live, and even if I did, they predicted that I would never talk or walk again. The term in the '80s was 'vegetable', a label that nobody chooses. After my accident, my personality became extroverted and socially inappropriate. It was difficult for me to engage emotionally, and I trusted everyone. My ability to distinguish between good and not-so-good people was non-existent for years after my accident, and I had to relearn how to do everything. I am still learning, but my filter for sorting this information has improved.

The people referred to in this book are mostly referenced by first name only because some of them are not a part of my life anymore, and I do not know if they would want to be included in my story. One consequence of brain injury is that your friends and family, and all who knew you, need to relate to or even love a 'new you'–the person they once knew but can no longer recognise because you have changed. Your brain chemistry is now different, and injury to the brain can cause significant personality and behavioural changes on many levels. Not all of your friends will be able to cope with those changes. If you are caring for a person with a brain injury, there may also be people who walk away for their own reasons. In my case, many did walk away. For me, that was one of the hardest parts of the journey. Hope for something better kept me going.

I have summarised some of the key learning strategies at the end of each chapter (from Chapter 4) and included some proactive strategies at the end of this book. This will help manage many of the commonly experienced barriers and limitations that can result from a brain injury. These are strategies that have worked for me and for many of my clients within their occupational rehabilitation journeys. Acquired injuries result in having to navigate life differently and find the 'new you'. I promise that if you commit to improving your current situation and the challenges associated with brain injury by using the memory strategies and tips included in this book, you will increase your ability to reach your potential. My message is one of hope: hope that you will not give up trying to make the most of this precious life and that your best self will emerge, no matter the circumstances. When you hold on to hope, you can find a way. You can use the strategies in this book to enhance your life, and they will help you create the 'new you' on your own terms. Reading this book may be one of your first challenges in working towards improving your memory and concentration, so let's get started . . . one step at a time, or one page at a time.

Hit-and-run accident

A woman motor-cyclist, aged 16, is seriously ill in Christchurch Hospital after a hit-and-run accident at the corner of New Brighton Road and Bower Avenue last evening.

A police patrol car arrived at the scene soon after the accident, at 8 p.m., but the car that had been in the collision had already gone.

The police want to hear from anyone who has seen a green 1966 HR Holden, registration CV4048.

Chapter 1

How it Was

When my parents and I moved to New Zealand from Australia in 1974, we arrived as a family: my father, my mother and I. Dad had resigned from his secure and profitable job with a concreting firm in Brisbane to pursue deer culling work. He had learned of the opportunity from his mate John, who was also working as a deer culler. We moved to Fox Glacier on the west coast of the South Island of New Zealand when I was three years old. Dad had been born in New Zealand, and his family still lived there. He loved the deer culling work and did foot shooting for the NZ government when he was 17 years old. Mum did not realise how dangerous it was. The difference in deer culling in 1974 was the use of helicopters to hunt deer. In hindsight, she said that if she had known, she would never have agreed to the move. Nine months after relocating, Dad died in a tragic accident at work. He was 30 years old. Mum was left with no support in a foreign country. She was a 26-year-old woman with a three-year-old toddler. She was Australian-born, as was I. At the time, the welfare rules were much less generous for Australians in New Zealand than the reverse. As a single mother in New Zealand, she was not eligible for any welfare benefits because she was Australian and had not lived in NZ for the 12 years required to access Social Welfare.

She wrestled with the decision of whether to stay in New Zealand or go back to Australia. She decided to stay in New Zealand because of her belief that it was a better place to raise me. There was less crime, and it was a safer place to live. The consequences of that decision were hard, though. The result of not being able to access Social Welfare meant that Mum would work one full-time job and 1 or 2 part-time jobs. Sometimes there was not enough money to pay the electricity bill, or we had to live off soup. There were no luxury items such as a colour television or car until I was a teenager. Interest rates on home loans were 19% in the '70s, but we were lucky to have a secure roof over our heads. There was no shortage of love, but life was difficult. One of Mum's wage packets went to pay for my babysitters. She worked in low-paying jobs as a waitress, barmaid, cleaner, chairlift operator, and secretary. She was a young mum, and we had a close bond, born out of having only each other to rely on for many years. She knew that education was a way out of poverty, which was why she worked so many jobs to enrol me in quality schools where I would receive an excellent education. When Mum was 39 years old, she decided to fulfil her high school ambition and began training to become a registered nurse. She started her full-time nursing course at Polytech in 1987 while continuing to work part-time. This was now possible because she had become eligible for the widow's benefit when I turned 15. I am forever grateful for the work ethic Mum taught me and the excellent education I received.

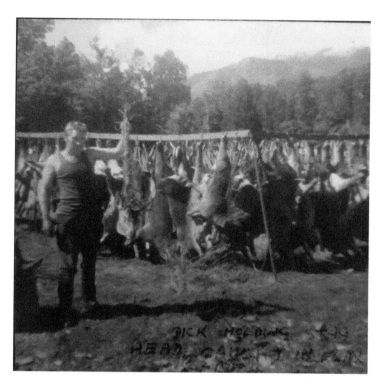

DICK HOLDING
HEAD

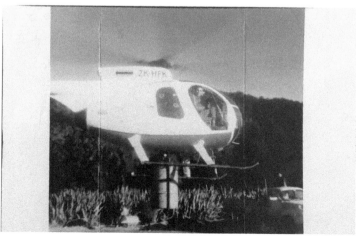

About a year after Dad's death, Mum decided to relocate to Christchurch. We lived in a small duplex in New Brighton, which Mum had purchased with a $5000 deposit. The funds provided through my Father's life insurance policy enabled this new start.

Our new neighbours, Audrey and Ivan, moved into the duplex next to us, and they became my surrogate grandparents. I would often rock up on their doorstep after school and sit with Audrey in her sewing room. Audrey was a dressmaker and made beautiful clothes. While she was working, I shared stories of my days at school, such as my first primary school crush on a boy called Chris. Ivan played my surrogate father at my debutante ball and gave me away at my wedding.

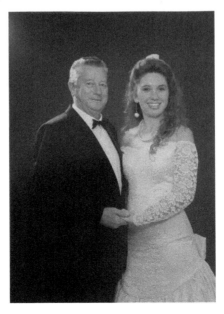

They became family. We lived in one of those neighbourhoods where we all knew each other by name, and we could walk into each other's houses without knocking. Many of the neighbours were elderly and watched us kids grow up. A family around the corner had six girls, and I started my first day of primary school with Ronda and Marie. We are still friends. We would play on grass islands in the middle of the road, and we had running races on them while our neighbours watched from their homes. Some of the neighbours babysat me over the years when Mum could not find a decent babysitter to care for me while she was at work. Mum's side of the family was all in Australia, and my father's family lived on the North Island.

When I was 16, I bought my first motorbike. I hung out with a great group of girls from my high school who identified with gothic music and clothing. Black became my staple wardrobe element, and I began to experiment with marijuana. I wanted to go to university and study psychology. My school reports suggested that I was not strongly focused on academics. Feedback from my teachers included statements such as, 'Nicole could achieve much better results with focus' or 'Easily distracted and not reaching the potential she has'. You get the drift. I was an average student who didn't try too hard but had the potential for more. Our limited financial resources also meant that it was unlikely that I could go to university.

Remember when you were 16 years old--pushing your boundaries, figuring out who you were, and thinking you were invincible? That was me. Fit, active, and challenging the imposed boundaries. Mum found it difficult to discipline me, and she was working 20 hours per week on top of her full-time nursing training. With assignments and study to complete, she was very busy. I was a wilful child, and I ignored my mother's warnings on that cold June night in 1987 when she insisted that I not take my motorbike out. She said she had a 'feeling' that something bad was going to happen. She had been saying similar things all week about a bad feeling she was having. With my teenage, 'know-it-all' attitude, my response to this was, 'Yeah right, Mum!' I did not take her seriously, and I just wanted to play basketball on that fateful night. My life was about to change forever. Mum seemed to know it, but I did not.

Earlier in the week, a thoughtful neighbour had brought over some beautiful purple and pink dried flowers to cheer Mum up. Mum had been feeling down and overwhelmed with everything she had on her plate. She could not shake the feeling that the flowers were a precursor to something ominous.

Chapter 2

A Once in a Lifetime Purchase

Father Time

It all started on one foreseen day,
After that, we were all left in total dismay.
The end of a beginning, the beginning of an end
Something the doctors thought impossible to
mend
But as we wait in frozen rhyme,
My mother kept saying, 'just wait for old
Father Time.'

Meanwhile, another steep hill to conquer would
appear,
And I'd pop another pill and say another
prayer.
This is all enough to drive any sane person
around the bend,
While with a look of horror,
I'd turn around and think, 'where is a friend?'

They were nowhere to be seen
And I wondered if they'd ever been,
But my mother kept saying, 'just wait for old
Father Time.'
As sympathy was mistaken for sorrow,
I simply began to hate the thought of tomorrow.

Although 'old Father Time' took the high road

And the low road to walk his slow mile,
The remainder spreads across my face
In a slow but joyous smile.

Nicole Yeates, 1990

I was in Form 6 at an excellent high school, and Mum's work ethic was already rubbing off on me. I had been working in some capacity since I was 12 years old. I had part-time jobs, including babysitting and bakery work, but when I was 15, I got a job with a company called Nurse Maude. I worked there during school holidays as a home support worker for the elderly. I cleaned their houses and did their shopping and other errands to help keep them independent in their own homes. I loved the work and the money. During the school term, I did the milk run. I woke up at 4:45 am to start work and ran through the streets pushing cartons of milk on a trolley. We delivered door-to-door, which took around 1 ½ hours. I earned $5 for each delivery shift. I would then cycle to school on my push-bike. After school, I attended hockey or netball practise at least once per week. I also played competitive netball and hockey on the weekend. I was so fit and healthy!

I got my first tax refund at age 16, and it was a grand total of $175.00. It was not enough to buy a car, but it was enough to buy a motorbike, pay for my licence, and buy myself some new jeans. Mum was horrified! She forbade me to get the bike. With teenage indignation I told her, 'It is my money, and I can do what I want with it!' In New Zealand, you could get your driver's licence at age 15. So, after a look through the local newspaper, I found a Suzuki 50CC bike for sale for $100. I did not know how to ride a motorbike, but what the hell, I would learn. I was invincible, right? So, during March 1987, I wandered down to the seller's house (while Mum was at work), which was about a 20-minute walk, and I made the purchase. The seller gave me a helmet with the bike, but it was too big, and it was not a full-face helmet. He gave me a brief lesson on how to operate the motorcycle, but I did not have a licence yet, so I walked the bike home. Oh yes, I was determined!

Mum arrived home from work to find that I had bought the motorbike. With one look at the helmet, she knew it was useless, and she insisted on buying me a top-notch, full-face helmet. She also insisted that I complete a Safe Motorcycle Riding course. Sensible steps indeed! The helmet she purchased for me cost more than the bike! I learned how to ride it in our backyard, initially. After all, I had to know how to ride the bike to take the course. I completed the course, and I relegated my bicycle to the garage while I exercised my 16-year-old freedom on my new motorbike.

I got my licence, and because I was the equivalent of a learner driver, I was not permitted to carry pillion passengers. Another rule to break, and quickly. Within two weeks of having the bike, I visited my friend Bridget after school. We went to Marian College in Christchurch. Bridget asked me for a ride on my bike, so why not? She got onto the back of my bike. We only got about 50 metres before toppling onto the sidewalk grass in fits of giggles. Bridget thought she was too fat, but we were 16, and I think most of us thought we were too fat. We were not fat. I was not strong enough to manage a bike and a pillion passenger. That was the first minor accident. Then there was a second one. This was not really an accident but an incident that should have served as a warning. A young student at the boys' high school across from our Catholic, girls-only high school lived in the same suburb and worked in the local shop, which was owned by his parents. He asked me for a ride home from school. Why not? Between amnesia and the 33 years that have passed, I cannot be sure of his name, but I think it was Dwayne. Dwayne was a tall and solid lad, and I found him to be cheerful and personable. He climbed on the back of my bike, and as I sped up, the weight of this pillion passenger caused the front of my bike to lift in the air. I had just done my first 'wheelie'! We laughed and thought we were cool. I accelerated more cautiously for the remainder of the 15-minute run back to his parents' shop.

Amnesia is a strange thing to live with. Retrograde amnesia is when a person loses the ability to remember part or all of their past, while anterograde amnesia is when a person loses memories after a particular event. In more severe cases, a person loses sections of memory from both before *and* after the event. That is what happened to me. I have a recollection of some memories. My early childhood is reasonably clear. For example, I recall helping Dad clean the outside of our house in Fox Glacier when I was three years old. That is my only conscious memory of him. I remember objecting strongly to Mum's attempt to dissuade me from taking my bike out on that cold June night in 1987. The two to three years before my accident and the two to three years after are hazy. Mum assures me that I went to a Dire Straits concert about 12 months after my accident. I went with friends of hers, but I have absolutely *zero* memory of that. Apparently, I had a great time! To enable me to write this book, the gaps in my memory have been filled in by my mum, by documents written during my time in a coma, by medical reports, and by friends and family.

Before my motorcycle accident, I was a good judge of character. I was a little introverted--the sort of person who would go to a party and only mingle with the people I knew because I was not confident enough to go beyond that socially. I felt awkward. Sixteen is an awkward age for most people. My mother tells me I was a loving and affectionate child, and I know I had respect for my elders. I was the kind of young lady who stood up on a bus when adults were standing. Mum raised me with good values, and I had never really gotten into any major trouble.

On the night of Friday, 19 June 1987, it was cold, rainy, and dark. I had plans to play basketball with my friend Maree, and some of our girlfriends from high school were coming to watch. The cold and rain seemed to enhance my mother's sense of dread. She asked me to call one of my friends who had a car to see if they could pick me up, and she relayed her fear that something bad was going to happen.

I refused to call, so Mum called my friend Lisa and asked her if I could get a ride with her. Mum did not own a car because the cost was beyond her resources. Lisa agreed to pick me up and bring me home after the basketball game. I objected strongly and refused to accept this help. Mum called Lisa back and told her that I had refused her offer. Public transport was terrible back then, and I would have had to get two buses to reach the basketball venue, which would have taken at least 2 hours just to get there, as the bus service at night was not very good. I was determined to take my bike and just would not listen to Mum. I agreed to drive to Lisa's and go from there to basketball in her car. Mum continued to try to convince me to accept the ride from Lisa and to change my jacket from the dark one I was wearing to a lighter-coloured one to increase my visibility. Determined to assert my independence and not acknowledging Mum's sense of foreboding, I stomped my feet and told her, 'I am 16 and can do what I want!' With that, I rushed out of the house and jumped on my motorbike.

I drove off into the dark, focused on playing basketball and seeing my friends. It was meant to be an enjoyable night with the girls. As I drove along Avon Avenue, I was rugged up in winter wear and was wearing my top-notch, full-face helmet.

Mum remained deeply concerned and felt helpless. It would normally have taken me around 20 minutes to drive to Lisa's house. Mum waited for 45 minutes before ringing Lisa again, as she still had not heard from me. Lisa told her that I had not yet arrived. Panic set in. Mum knows that I am ALWAYS on time. I am never late for anything! After an hour, Mum called the hospitals. Nothing. No news. She phoned the police to find out if there had been any accidents. Nothing. In desperation, she phoned Lisa again, and by this time Lisa was also worried. Lisa agreed to follow the route I would take to get to her place, down Avon Avenue, to see if perhaps I was stranded due to my bike breaking down again. There were no mobile phones in those days!

The road was quiet. The night was dark, and I was approaching a roundabout. I was not speeding, but as I approached the intersection of the roundabout, the lights on my motorbike went out. I was suddenly riding in the dark, and since I could not stop in the middle of the roundabout, I planned to get to the other side and try to figure out what had gone wrong with my lights. Since buying my motorbike, I had learned to change my spark plugs and various other minor mechanical bits and pieces, so I hoped I could figure it out. That opportunity never came.

I do not remember being hit by the green Ford Falcon; however, witnesses informed the police of what happened after the car ran me down.

A man in his early twenties was driving the vehicle. He did not see me, but there can be no doubt that he heard and felt the impact of the collision with my motorbike. He kept driving. Witnesses reported that my motorbike became entangled in his vehicle's bumper bar. They stated that sparks were flying, and the bike eventually caught fire. I had become entangled in the bike. He dragged my youthful body and the motorcycle on the cold, hard road for hundreds of metres before I was disentangled and set free from the vicious impact. My bike remained attached to his bumper bar. He continued driving for approximately one kilometre before my bike detached itself, and when it did, it took his licence plate with it. He did not offer himself to police following the accident.

The local newspaper, The Star, advertised for information to identify this hit-and-run driver, and police were able to track him down. We will never know if he was drunk or not, but we do know he was unlicenced. The police found his car's licence plate on the side of the road the next day and were able to find him.

He left me for dead in the middle of the road. As luck would have it, a nurse from the local spinal unit at Burwood Hospital happened to be driving by. Mark was travelling alone in his car when he noticed what looked like a jacket in the middle of the road, and he pulled over to pick it up. What he found was me. Mark had oxygen in his car. He ensured that my spine was stable, cleared my airway, and kept me breathing on oxygen whilst calling an ambulance. By this time a crowd had gathered, and they were praying on the side of the road. Because of the rain and a higher incidence of accidents, the ambulance would take another 30 minutes to reach me. In the meantime, Mark kept me alive.

Chapter 3

My Near-Death Experience

The police arrived at Mum's house whilst I was still on the road. She saw the blue and red lights flashing through the front window of the house. The police officer's footsteps pounded the footpath, and Mum could hear him as he approached the front door. Her heart sank–she just knew. He knocked. She answered the door, and before they said anything, she stammered, 'It's Nicole, isn't it? Is she ok?' The police officer informed her that there had been a hit-and-run accident, and I was seriously injured. He advised her that they should go straight to the hospital. She felt numb. Mum wanted to go to the accident scene, but she was told by the officer that the ambulance was probably already at the hospital. He recommended that they go straight there. She walked to the police car, and they began the drive to Christchurch Public Hospital. As they were driving, Mum uttered to the police officer, *'God would not take Nicole from me as he knows that that would be too much for me to bear.'* He kept driving. What could he say?

As they continued towards the hospital, Mum asked the policeman to go back to our house after he dropped her off. She wanted him to remove the pink and purple flowers from our house or speak with our neighbours about removing them. She acknowledged that her thoughts about this were irrational, but she also felt that if the flowers remained in the house, I would not be coming home. To the officer's credit, he went back and removed the flowers for her. It was a touching act of human kindness, for which she was most grateful.

My friends, Lisa and Maree drove past the accident site, near the Avon River bridge, and saw that the police were there. They knew instinctively that it was me. They got out of the car and nervously walked up to an officer, who told them that a girl on a motorcycle had been in an accident. Although the officer did not mention my name, they knew it was me. Lisa recalls that she and Maree drove to my house to let Mum know, but she had already left when they arrived. They went back to Lisa's house to tell Lisa's parents, Sandy and Paul, what had happened, and Lisa's parents drove them to the hospital.

Mum arrived at the hospital before I did. She was beside herself with fear and dread. Would Nicole be alive on arrival? Was she ok? Was she in pain? She waited and prayed.

Back at the scene of the accident, Mark remained with me. He had already administered resuscitation. My arms were rigidly bent up to my chest in a tonic spasm, indicating a major brain or spinal injury. My left arm would remain tightly held to my chest like this for many weeks. Finally, the ambulance arrived. As the ambulance officers prepared to move me into the ambulance, Mark corrected their method of transferring me. This action would prevent further permanent paralysis if a spinal injury were present. The ambulance rushed me to the hospital.

At the hospital, the policeman announced to Mum that the ambulance had arrived. Mum rushed toward the accident & emergency room. I was groaning–a loud, guttural, unnatural sound of pain personified. She yelled out to let me know she was there. 'I am here, honey. Fight, please fight!'

I was covered in blood; my eyeballs were rolling, and she could see the whites of my eyes. My left eye was black, and I smelled of petrol. The medical team worked quickly, their movements rapid and focused. Mum looked to the doctors and nurses for reassurance, but they turned away. They had nothing to say, but the looks on their faces said it all. Mum sensed my father's presence around me. I began to vomit; I was bringing up bile from my stomach. The medical team rushed me to a CT scan. Mum was holding my hand and running with the medical team. Suddenly they told Mum to leave, and the curtains closed. Mum had my blood all over her.

Our neighbours, Audrey and Ivan, had now arrived, and they saw what was happening before the curtains in the CT room closed. The medical team had the defibrillator on me as the paddles of life were in action.

I heard the doctor say, 'We've lost her; she's gone.' I remember stating, 'No you bloody haven't!'

I could see myself above the trolley at the CT scanner. The doctors did not seem to hear me when I was speaking. The next thing I remember is seeing a yellow light. I had a sense of peace beyond any words I know. I was in a space that felt beautiful, harmonious, safe, and secure. It was harmony filled with a powerful feeling of love. I felt embraced by it, and I surrendered for a moment to enjoy the blissful tranquillity. I had forgotten the doctors' words and their belief that I was gone. I saw my father. He was wearing a smart black suit with a black tie. He was still 30 years old, and he said to me, 'C'mon, Sassafras.'

I was invited to go with him—to be with my father. I said to Dad, 'No. What about Mum? She needs me.' I turned away, but it was hard because this place was so beautiful, and I loved my father too.

Then I heard a voice. It was a deep voice; the voice of a man. It was the light speaking. It was not my father; he had gone. It was the light, the spirit. He did not introduce himself; he did not need a name. He said to me, 'Your time on earth is not done. You have more to teach.' I had questions, but I did not ask them. I was told about his plan. I was told that it does not matter if we go to church or not. Churches were never part of the plan. He never wanted a multitude of different religions. What matters is how we live, that we are good people, and it need not be any more complicated than that.

I had been educated in Catholic schools and was familiar with the concept of heaven and hell. They taught me that if you were not a good person, you would go to hell. The tenets of the church have a strong tendency to 'persuade' that as a Catholic, you should go to church. There is judgement that if you do not, you are not a 'good Catholic'. I was surprised to hear this alternative information from the spirit but also relieved. I was more convinced by his spirit words than I had ever been by anyone involved in my Catholic education!

When I was in the CT scanner, Ivan (who was waiting outside with Mum) heard a member of the medical team say to the doctor who worked on me in death, 'You've done a wonderful job!' I had experienced cardiac arrest, but my heart was now beating again. Audrey and Ivan were comforting each other, and Mum continued to wait.

Mum was still waiting outside, too scared to look or listen. A female doctor approached her and knelt in front of her to make direct eye contact. She said, 'I'm sorry, but expect death.' Frozen by these words, she could not move, think, or even cry. If she let her guard down . . . it was overwhelming to consider the consequences. Mum started to pray out loud.

The medical team ran again, and Mum ran with them. I was taken to the Intensive Care Unit (ICU), where my heart would stop beating again, and once again they would resuscitate me. I was placed on life support. They made Mum stay in the waiting room again, where she had an unknown visitor. The hospital priest had arrived to read me my last rites. Mum has described getting a terrible feeling from this man; she sensed evil, and his words did not help. He believed I was going to die, and he tried to convince Mum of this too. Audrey and Ivan were consoling each other. Mum was alone and consumed with fear. She continued to pray.

Mum needed support, too, but was feeling as alone as anyone can feel. She called Father Pat Crawford, who was the priest from my second primary school. He had become a family friend over the years and had shared many meals at our home. It was now around 10:30 pm, and he had been asleep when she rang. He came to the hospital straightaway. She also called my closest friend, Maree, and asked her to come. Mum was not aware yet that Lisa and her parents, Sandy and Paul, were in the waiting room on the other side of the hospital. Maree came back to the hospital. Mum then called her sister Carol in Australia. Carol reassured her that whilst I was sleeping in my coma, I was healing. Mum wanted to call her mother-in-law, but Nana had recently had a stroke, and Mum feared what the news could do to her.

When Mum could finally see me, I was in the ICU and connected to life support. I had burn marks on my chest from the defibrillator and scratches and burns on my lower legs. The deep cut on my head had been closed with stitches. I was lying on my right side and looked as if I were sleeping, but there were multiple tubes and machines attached to me. Machines were breathing for me and keeping my heart beating. Sandy and Paul offered some comfort and support to Mum. Mum and Sandy realised that they already knew each other from work at the Burwood spinal unit. Maree came into my hospital room and fainted when she saw me. However, Mum was grateful to have her there, and once Maree gathered herself, she asked about what the doctors had said regarding my outlook. Father Crawford arrived and reassured Mum. They began to pray by my bedside, and they stayed all night. Mum could still feel Dad around us.

The medical team diagnosed me with a severe traumatic brain injury (TBI) with diffuse brain damage, which means damage to multiple areas of the brain. My left parietal skull bone was fractured, and there was damage to my brain stem, which regulates breathing and heart rate. The neurosurgeon told Mum that I had a 30 percent chance of survival. If I did survive, they expected me to remain in a vegetative state with paralysis. However, they could not sway her from her belief that I would recover. Over the next couple of days, doctors and nurses came to my bedside to do their tests and reassess my level of coma. I was unresponsive, and no reflexes were present. On day four of my coma, the neurosurgeon undertook the doll's eye test to assess my level of brain function. The doll's eye reflex tests brain stem function in comatose patients. Doll's eye means that when the head is moved from side to side, the eyes remain fixed in one position. It is an indicator of brain death. Mum recalls overhearing the doctor say, 'doll's eye', but she did not know what it meant. They would perform this test multiple times in the coming days.

The medical team recommended switching off my life support. Mum refused to allow it. She told them, 'You do not know my daughter. You do not know her spirit. You do not know how strong she is!' The medical team recommended further review of ongoing life support if my condition deteriorated, and they started a conversation about organ donation if the worst happened. Mum refused to engage in this discussion and remained firm in her conviction that I would survive.

Chapter 4

Yeates or Yates?

On the same night as my accident, a young man was also admitted to hospital following a motorcycle accident. Timothy Yates was two years older than me. His last name is pronounced the same as mine but spelled differently. Timothy had a severe brain injury and had to have one of his legs amputated. Like me, he was given a 30 percent chance of survival, and Mum and the Yates family become supporters of each other. Timothy and I were in beds next to each other in the ICU.

Mum stayed at the hospital all that first night but had to leave at 8:00 am. The staff told her that she could come back after 10:00 am when the doctors had finished their rounds. One of our neighbours picked her up from the hospital and took her home, so she could get changed and have a shower. Three of our neighbours came over while Mum was home, and they remained in the duplex while she freshened up and gathered her thoughts. They would tell her later that they stayed because they were afraid that she would harm herself if something happened to me. They remained close by. Father Crawford went home to take care of his community commitments. He came back the next day and anointed me again. By this time, the hospital staff had arranged for a bed near the ICU for Mum to stay in for a few nights. The only time she was not near my bedside was during the doctors' rounds in the morning.

The hospital priest continued to drop in unexpectedly. He seemed to appear out of nowhere. Mum continued to get a bad feeling about this man, and he distressed more than comforted her. The nursing staff appeared to pick up on this, and they would move closer to Mum when he came in. During one of these random visits, the priest gave Mum a rosary ring and declared it would help her with her prayers. She experienced bad vibes from the ring, so she threw it out the hospital window. Mum asked the nurses to let the priest know that she did not want him to visit again. She did not see him again after that.

On 20 June 1987, the day after my accident, the doctors examined me again. My withdrawal response to pain was not localising, corneal reflexes were not present, and there was no vocal response. Later that night, my medical record shows doll's eye negative, meaning that my brain stem was not intact.

By Sunday, 21 June 1987, news of my accident had filtered through to my Australian family (Mum's six brothers and sisters). Uncle Geoff still remembers the sense of urgency he felt to get on a plane and come to New Zealand to support us. Geoff had been working in the bush for many years and had never needed a driver's licence. Uncle Geoff had lived with us in Christchurch when I was about nine years old, and he knew the challenges with public transport, so he got a driver's licence before he came to New Zealand. A few days later, he arrived from Australia. He was heartbroken about my situation but became a significant support for both of us. Geoff watched Mum with admiration as she talked to me, trying to encourage me to open my eyes, constantly letting me know I was loved, and watching my eyes move back and forth under my eyelids as if they were looking for a way out. He took this eye movement as a sign of hope that my situation would improve. With Geoff now there to share the load, he encouraged Mum to go home and get some rest. Mum and Geoff alternated 12-hour shifts, so I was never left alone. I remained comatose in the ICU with Timothy.

Mum arrived home to an empty house. She went into my room and cried. What would become of her daughter? Her mind raced with all of the heartbreaking information and dire predictions from the medical team. The fear was overwhelming when she considered leaving me alone, even though she knew that I was not alone because Geoff was taking care of me. The risk that I could die was still high. Above the piano in our lounge room hung a family portrait of Mum, Dad, and me, which had been taken about 18 months before Dad's death. Ivan noticed that Mum was home and came over to check on her. As he walked in the door, he saw Mum hitting the photo above the piano. She was yelling at Dad, 'You can't take her!' Dad's presence was so strong that it created more fear in her. Our neighbours and friends continued to drop by the hospital to show their support, including a lovely lady who had employed me to look after her children. Deborah had three beautiful children, two girls and a boy, whom I had cared for regularly. They were easy kids to look after. Deborah was a religious woman. She announced to Mum that God had sent her a message for me: John 15, verse 7, 'If you remain in me and my words remain in you, ask whatever you wish, and it will be done for you.' Deborah reported her belief that I would walk out of that hospital. Mum clung onto those words with all her might!

On 22 June 1987, I convulsed. My brain injury had caused epilepsy. My seizures lasted 30–60 minutes, and the doctors added anti-seizure medication to my intravenous line. The examination on 23 June, showed no spontaneous eye opening, but my hospital notes state, 'Corneal, Doll's eye, trach reflex present'. On 24 June, the medical team decided that it was time to test whether I could breathe on my own. They expected the worst but hoped for the best. An ICU staff member approached Mum with some paperwork. Again, Mum had a nurse communicating with her about donating my organs. The nurse was empathetic, but Mum would not engage in that conversation. She told them yet again of her belief that her daughter's spirit was strong, and she would walk out of the hospital. She refused to sign the organ donation forms. The nurse looked at her with sadness because Mum could not accept their prediction that I could not survive such a catastrophic brain injury. Mum knew in her heart that I could hear her and feel her touch, even though there was no evidence of this from a medical point of view.

That spirit Mum spoke of came to the fore now, and when they turned off life support, I began to breathe on my own. I remained in a coma and on oxygen, and I was still considered critical. The medical team extubated me to remove the breathing support. I remained stable, and approximately eight days into my coma, the decision was made to move me out of the ICU and into the high dependency unit. Timothy and I seemed to remain on par, and they also moved him into the room with me. We both remained on oxygen, still critical, and were positioned in a room next to the nurses' station. We both remained unresponsive and in deep comas. There was a sense that only one of us would live through this, but both families hoped for the best and continued to support each other. Timothy's Uncle Andrew regularly visited him, and he became a tremendous support for Mum. Our friendship with Andrew and his son Rupert continued for years after.

Weeks went by, and I received many visitors. My school friends, our neighbours, friends, and people from our past who we had not seen for a long time visited the hospital or sent cards of support. Mum and Geoff tried everything to stimulate me out of that coma. They talked to me, and they played my favourite music (even my Violent Femmes music, which Mum hated!). Nothing worked. I responded to nothing. There was no sign of life or any evidence that I could hear them. Mum tried bribery. She promised to buy me a dog if I came out of the coma. We had a beautiful dog named Tammy when I was four years old, but she died three years later after being hit by a car. Because of financial strain, another dog had been out of the question. Mum knew how much I wanted a dog, and she hoped this promise would inspire me to wake up. I did not respond.

In further attempts to awaken me, Mum investigated alternative therapies. One of our neighbours had a daughter who was a homeopath. Homeopathy supports the theory that natural resources can treat illness, and the body can heal itself. The natural remedies are chosen to trigger the body's natural defences. This homeopath spoke with Mum about Bach Flower Rescue Remedy and Arnica, which she believed would assist. Some theories about these natural remedies include that it will strengthen a person's willpower, aid stress management, restore calm, and provide relief of pain, inflammation, and reduce bruising. Mum was desperate for me to wake up. The longer I remained in a coma, the worse the prognosis became. She began to put a few drops of Bach Flower Rescue Remedy under my tongue a few times per day. She did not tell the medical team she was doing this.

During the first week of July, Timothy and I were moved out of the high dependency unit and into ward 12B. We had our own rooms now, but they adjoined. When Timothy's family was not in the room with him, Mum monitored him too. Timothy's father had died from cancer some 18 months earlier, and his mum, sisters, Uncle Andrew, and extended family often visited. Mum got to know Timothy through his family. Andrew and Mum would sometimes go to the hospital chapel together and pray for us both. On Sunday, 5 July 1987, Timothy Yates lost his battle for survival and was pronounced dead. A young man in the prime of his life, with a bright future ahead of him, had had his time cut short. The sadness and grief were raw. Although fear had never left, it was further ignited about my situation. Both families had held so much hope that we would both make it out of the hospital alive. The Yates family remained supportive of Mum despite their grief as they made plans for Timothy's funeral.

They buried Timothy on 7 July 1987, and it was on that day that I opened my eyes for the first time. This was 19 days from the date of my accident. My eyes did not remain open, and the doctor said it was a reflex reaction. Seeing my eyes open gave Mum and Geoff hope. The doctors were not as optimistic. Timothy's family returned from having buried their handsome young man and visited with Mum. How brave they were to share in the happiness of me opening my eyes after enduring such tragedy and sadness themselves on that day. Mum felt a mixture of emotions: hope because I had opened my eyes and guilt because I had survived and Timothy had not. Sadness and fear still lurked, but hope was to be the emotion that sustained her.

KEY LEARNINGS

- Stimulation during coma is important to help your loved one know that they are supported, and there is also evidence that stimulation during a coma can improve oromotor dysfunction (Roig-Quilis, 2015). The oromotor system includes feeding, nutrition, articulation, and gestural non-verbal communication. Although studies have shown that formal sensory stimulation programs for persons in a coma may not be sufficient to restore consciousness, they can increase arousal and improve oromotor function (Cheng et al., 2018).

- Helpful actions during the coma phase, as advised by my mother (who did all of these things) include:

  Use massage therapy.

  Ensure constant verbal, auditory, and sensory stimuli throughout the day, such as speaking to them, reading books to them, and playing music.

  Introduce passive exercises (especially feet and contractured limbs) as early as possible. Physiotherapists can show you what to do.

  Research natural therapies to complement medical therapies.

  Engage friends and family to provide stimuli while they are visiting.

Utilise a visitors' book and get the visitors to document in the book any changes they see from visit to visit.

Chapter 5

My Slow Awakening

I gradually awakened from my coma over the next few weeks. I am told that there were periods when I had my eyes open, but I was still considered to be in a semi-comatose state. I initially could not see and was unable to move, unable to talk, and had no control of my bodily functions. Mum continued to believe I was going to walk and talk again. As if to prove a point, the medical team removed me from my bed using a hoist and placed me in a wheelchair. I could not move any part of my body, and my left arm remained contracted to my chest. I had also developed foot drop from being unconscious for so long. My head had to be held up by a halo connected to the wheelchair. Mum was told, 'This is the way it may always be.'

Mum, Geoff, and my visitors continued to stimulate me both when I was sleeping and during my 'awake' periods. I would sometimes respond to commands, but this was inconsistent.

Still, Mum was determined. She had to defer her nursing studies to care for me, and she set about trying to prove that I had some element of cognition left in my brain. It started with simple instructions–trying to awaken me, asking me to blink, those sorts of things. My sight returned, and my brain was starting to engage.

I still could not walk or talk; I remained catheterised and had a nasogastric tube for feeding. I had some limited use of my left hand. Mum brought a notepad into the hospital to see if I could communicate in writing. My writing resembled that of a three-year-old, but it was a start. For my first communication, I wrote, 'Where is my dog?!' I had been listening whilst in a coma!

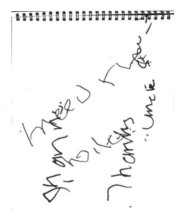

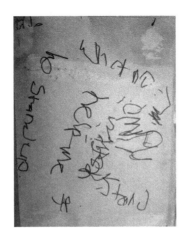

I had reverted to about the age of a three-year-old functionally as well. Mum started trying to get me to do things for myself, such as brush my hair. Attempts at verbal communication were brief, sometimes comprehensible, and when I did start to verbally communicate, I spoke rapidly in a high-pitched voice. I babbled inappropriate things. I had little strength, but I could sometimes raise my right arm to my head with a brush, on command. The action was not me brushing my hair, but it was me trying, and I could do it once but not repeatedly. It was something, however, and that little 'something' enhanced hope. At this stage, I had only managed to perform this action in front of Mum. The doctors continued to believe that Mum was in denial, and they advised her that my responses were more 'reflex actions'–a phrase she was getting so sick of hearing! When she asked me to do the brush action in front of a doctor, I did! The doctor said it was 'just a reflex.' But when I felt fatigued, which was most of the time, my cognition was inconsistent. The doctor remained unconvinced that it was a purposeful, cognitive response.

I was awake enough to sit in a wheelchair but still needed a halo attached to hold up my head. Mum or Geoff would take me on brief excursions to a lovely park near the hospital. These outings were to increase my stimulation and enjoy some sunshine and fresh air. On our way out of the hospital on one of these excursions, Mum remembers passing a nun as she wheeled me along.

The nun said, 'Veronica, there are always miracles, but they are usually slow miracles.' At the time, she did not realise how true this would be.

Thirty-nine days postinjury, I began to bear weight with the assistance of two people, and I was communicating more. I was having longer periods of wakefulness, and I revealed many secrets to my mother, which I never would have done while of sound mind. You know, those naughty things you got up to as a teenager that your parents were never meant to find out about! These secrets included my recent first experience with marijuana. I also told Mum how I had carried pillion passengers on my motorbike when I was not supposed to. The most troubling secret was the sexual assault I had experienced as a seven-year-old. My inner voice remained an open book for many months. My sentences were incomplete, but long-term memories were unravelling. I remained on oxygen and still had a catheter. Keeping me on oxygen was something new that the medical team was trialling to improve brain injury outcomes. A current review of the literature for the use of oxygen after initial emergency treatment in improving outcomes for TBI patients is not convincing. What is known is that maintaining oxygen levels above 90% can help reduce secondary brain injury and reduce swelling in the brain. About six weeks postinjury, they took my gastric tube out, but I remained on oxygen and was still catheterised. They also took my IV line out.

Although I was now tolerating oral food, my mind and my stomach were frequently out of sync. I would get a craving for Kentucky Fried Chicken and beg one of my friends to sneak it into the hospital. By the time they got the food to me, I could not eat it because I was not feeling hungry or had forgotten I had even asked for it. Another craving Lisa vividly remembers me requesting frequently was Coke. Mostly, the food I got was hospital food. Not exactly an inspiring menu, but my brain had not regained all its autonomic functions yet. I still had no bladder control, my temperature regulation was inconsistent, and my hunger responses were not reliably present.

My responses grew more consistent throughout August, and I responded to more commands. Although my speech was slowly improving, I still had a long way to go. My friends still visited, and I could interact with them, although not always appropriately. I would say whatever came to my mind, and I could be offensive at times. My brain injury had removed the filter from my thought processes. If a visitor had gone to the trouble of carefully camouflaging the pimple on their face, I would point it out. If there was an inappropriate sexual connotation that could be applied to an innocent situation, I would state it. If I did not like someone, I would say so. There was also a nurse that I did not seem to like very much, and Mum tells me I would wet my bed on every one of her shifts! My behaviour would be a challenge for a long time.

Often, when visitors arrived at the hospital during those weeks after I had opened my eyes, they would find a sleeping Nicole. It did not take much to tire me in those early days. On one such occasion, Geoff wanted to talk about rehabilitation options during his visit with me, but I was sound asleep. Instead of waking me, he decided to leave me a letter. There was much to consider and many people to consult.

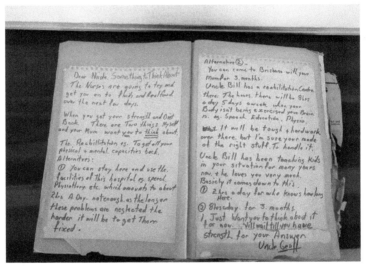

My formal rehabilitation started, and I began to walk, one awfully slow and painful step at a time. I went to physiotherapy in the hospital to build strength, work on my balance, and learn to walk again. I called them the 'monkey bars'–the physical therapy parallel bars used to assist people to walk. I had no coordination, left-sided hemiplegia, and foot drop, but I had a great physiotherapist who had not written me off as a lost cause. She was encouraging, and she pushed me when it all felt too hard. Mum and Geoff also encouraged me, and in between physio sessions, they would help me practise when the nurses were not watching.

There was another young man, two years older than me, who was also learning to walk again. His name was Andrew. Andrew had incurred a brain injury while bicycling home from his girlfriend's house one night, and he had also been in a coma. I do not recall the time we shared, re-learning to walk, but our paths would cross again outside of the hospital, and he would remember me.

Things were looking up, but my brain had not yet switched on in many regards, despite my consciousness. I remained on oxygen. My body still could not regulate my temperature normally, and I could not balance independently. After reliance on intravenous nutrients for so many weeks, I was underweight. My weight had dropped to 39 kg, a loss of 17 kg, but my brain was not telling me I was hungry. When food arrived, I often could not eat it. To 'manage' this, I would pack one side of my mouth with food and pretend to eat it. I would hide the food up my sleeves or under my bottom. I had to be force-fed until my brain's hunger response mechanism switched back on, which happened around 12 months later.

The lack of bladder control was humiliating when visitors were present. I would sometimes sit in the hospital bed when friends were visiting, not realising I had urinated in my bed. I could not tell I had wet myself until I felt the wetness on my skin. This was a consequence of paralysis. I would sit in my urine until my friends left. I have never asked them, but with more mature hindsight, I imagine that their senses of smell were much better than mine. The stench of my urine probably encouraged their departure at times. Although I could bear weight, it took a large amount of concentration to get my legs to move. There were still areas of my body that were paralysed. My mind was still confused, and I did not remember most of what had happened to me or many of the details of my life before the accident.

Around the beginning of August, it was time for Geoff to return to his fiancée and his work in Australia. He had been a champion. Geoff kept me company, encouraged me, told me jokes, massaged my rigid limbs, and supported both Mum and me in this journey towards a new 'normality'. He was so patient. It was lucky that Mum had a big family, with six brothers and sisters. The next sibling to cross the ditch was my Uncle Bill, Mum's eldest brother. Bill had a Master's in special education and worked as a special needs teacher. His skills would be well-utilised and appreciated in my recovery process.

I continued to work in the gym and in hydrotherapy daily and improved rapidly. In the water, I had more mobility, and I improved my strength and coordination. Around the beginning of August, Mum started her campaign to bring me home, but there were a few tests I had to pass first. The doctors were understandably concerned that Mum might not be able to manage me on her own.

I still needed help to get to the toilet, and I feared the dark because my balance was worse in the dark. I could not get myself up from a seated or lying position. Does going home sound ambitious?

Concerns aside, I had Mum and her friend Cos on my side. Cos was a physiotherapist from the Burwood Hospital spinal unit. Mum and Cos had met whilst Mum was doing volunteer work at the spinal unit before she started her nursing studies. Cos had invented a huge tricycle to help spinal injury patients. She believed that it would help increase my body movement and strength. They decided it was time to bring the bike into the hospital. Cos must have had to do some passionate negotiating and use her connections, but they agreed to trial the tricycle, and it was moved into ward 12B. The doctors had their doubts, and the hospital physiotherapists were watching intently. They did not think I could operate the tricycle. The goal was to prove that my coordination was improving, and they should consider me for hospital release. It was a tentative time. No one knew if I could do it, but they sure had loads of encouragement and hope.

Getting me onto the bike was a process, but once I was on it, I made those wheels turn with an enormous smile on my face! There were cheers of joy, and I felt a freedom I hadn't experienced since awakening. I rode around the ward, feeling rather proud. Mum and Cos were beaming. The first test was done. The hospital physios were astounded. They could not believe how quickly

I was progressing. Little did they know that Cos and Mum had me practising on that bike in the evenings when no one was around. They also had me practising the other tests I would need to pass to get medical approval to go home.

The next test was the stair test. I had to be able to walk up and down 3–4 stairs. Mum had me practising this day and night. There were lots of slip-ups, but eventually, I could do it.

The final test was the balance test. I had to be able to stand with my eyes closed, and I had to be able to take steps independently. I had to maintain balance if pushed (without the support of a wall or chair or person). This is the test I remember most vividly. The neurosurgeon came to the hospital room. He did not glow with warmth but was doing his job in the clinical manner that most surgeons share. I was determined. I now had my mind set on getting back home, and I willingly shared this information with anyone who would listen. I was intent on 'proving the doctors wrong'! Mum and I had been practising, just as we did with everything else, but I had been secretly practising on my own too! I pass the 'walking independently without falling over' test. I pass the 'standing with eyes closed' test. Now for the big one. I was feeling like a block of concrete, and I had to be if I was going to pass this test! I was determined that this doctor would NOT push me over. He nudged me, but I remained firm. I passed the push test.

KEY LEARNINGS
- Carers can feel very helpless through the coma

phase, but the tips provided in the previous chapter can help them become more involved in the patient's recovery. When the patient becomes more alert, more active exercises can be introduced. My mother sought advice from the physiotherapists and learned which exercises would be most beneficial, and she spoke to friends and family about learning how to administer these exercises as well. I received administered exercise up to six times per day.

- If you have family and friends around, then there is an opportunity to share the workload. The person who is the main caregiver may not be in the headspace to reach out for help, but support can still be provided (with permission, of course) to arrange a roster of shifts so that the comatose patient gets maximum stimuli and care from friends and family who are able to participate.

- Encourage the patient to practise exercises outside of formal physiotherapy, psychology, occupational therapy, and other treatment-based appointments. The more effort a patient puts into their treatment recommendations, the higher the likelihood of positive improvements.

- Hydrotherapy is a very effective physiotherapy, as the water takes any pressure off painful or rigid limbs, allowing more movement.

NICOLE IS THE BRAVEST GIRL I KNOW & SOON, YOU'LL BE FEELING LOTS BETTER.

You MUST KEEP TURNING YOUR HEAD TO THE RIGHT OF YOUR BODY TO STRENGTHEN YOUR NECK MUSCLES BECAUSE AS SOON AS YOU GAIN STRENGTH IN YOUR HEAD MOVEMENTS, YOU WILL BE ABLE TO SIT IN A CHAIR & WILL BE ABLE TO GO TO THE TOILET!

WON'T THAT BE GREAT!

THEN YOU CAN GO TO PHYSIO AND DO GYM WORK FOR YOUR BODY TO GET BETTER

Chapter 6

Creating a New Reality

It was time to go home on a trial basis. They discharged me from hospital on 7 August 1987, but the doctors warned Mum not to expect too much. The clinical psychologist at the hospital told Mum not to expect me to finish high school. I was discharged with phenobarbitone, a medication to control my epilepsy. The medical team still did not have high hopes for me! The theme that I could never finish school, go to university, work in a meaningful role, etc. continued. It was a medical model of care that had kept me alive, but it would take more than that to exceed the medical professionals' low expectations.

Mum did not have a car, so we had to ride the bus home. With my now redeveloping brain, I would ramble much like a three-year-old rambles, often making little sense. I was still trying to make connections between the world around me and how it related to me. People often zoned out because I would go on and on. I would keep going on and on because my perception was no longer intact, and I did not notice the normal social cues when someone was disinterested or annoyed. On the bus ride home, I was waffling on about a yellow light. At first, Mum thought I was talking about the traffic lights, but I got her attention when I stated indignantly, 'No Mum. You know, the yellow light when I died!'

Mum asked, 'What did you see?'

'Oh, it was beautiful Mum, so peaceful and beautiful. I wanted to stay.'

'Why didn't you?'

'You needed me, Mum!'

She asked me, 'Was there anyone at the yellow light?'

'Yes', I replied. 'There was a man.'

'What did he look like?'

'He was tall, slim, handsome, and he had very short hair.'

'What was he wearing?'

Thoughtfully, I replied, 'Um, he was wearing a black suit, with a white shirt and black tie.'

I had just described my father and the clothes he had been buried in, but I had only been three years old when he died and had not been at his funeral. As I mentioned earlier, Mum could instinctively feel Dad around, but because I was still figuring out how all the bits of my life fit together, she did not want to fill in the gaps for me.

Mum continued to help me independently recall who this man was. She asked me, 'Did this man say anything to you, love?'

'Yes, Mum. He said, "Come on, Sassafras."'

The blood drained out of Mum's face. This was all the evidence she needed to know that her instincts were spot on. It was my father. Sassafras was a nickname Dad had called me as a baby, and he was the only person to ever call me that. Dad had a pet possum when he was a kid and called it Sassafras. The possum was cute and cuddly, and so was I as a baby–hence the correlation. Mum had never told me this. The only way I could have known was to speak with my father. I had not been called this since his death when I was three years old.

She remained silent for a while and then asked me, 'Was there anyone else at the yellow light?'

'Yes Mum, I saw Jesus.'

'What did he look like?'

I looked at Mum in disbelief at this question. 'He didn't "look" like anything, Mum! He was the light!'

'Oh, ok, sorry', she said. 'Did he say anything?'

'He shared so much. It was really interesting.'

'Like what?' Mum asked.

'He said that we don't need to go to church. Churches were never part of the plan. He said we just need to be good people. He said that it wasn't my time yet and that I had more to teach.'

'What does he want you to teach?'

'I am not sure Mum. I can't remember.'

She remained silent, thinking of all I had revealed. Our home was only about 200 metres from the bus stop. I ambled along with Mum supporting me. As we walked the pathway from the bus stop to our home, a path I had walked almost daily since I was five years old, I had no memory of this place. It was all new, a blank canvas.

Mum opened the front door to our home, and I cautiously walked in. I soon spied the portrait of our family above the piano. *'Mum! That's the man!'*

'What man, dear?'

'That man in the photo, that is *the man I saw at the yellow light!* That is him!'

'Do you know who he is?'

'No. Who is he?'

'That is your father.'

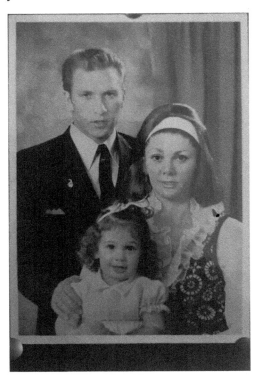

Mum showed me to my room. I liked my room. I opened my wardrobe, and there were many clothes. I asked Mum, 'Whose clothes are these?'

'They are your clothes, Nicole.'

Nothing was familiar. I disliked the black clothes in my wardrobe. I wanted to wear bright, colourful clothes.

It was time for dinner. I did not want to eat, and I could no longer get away with hiding my food (up my sleeves, in the sides of my wheelchair, etc.). Now that I was home, I made multiple trips to the toilet to dispose of the food in my mouth that I did not want. When you are not hungry, you simply do not want to eat. I needed forceful encouragement. Mum told me that there were many times when one meal would take up to three hours to feed me, as I would keep making excuses to leave the room. Uncle Bill was helpful to Mum when he came over to NZ for the 2 weeks and helped her with the feeding process. Basically, gave her a bit of a break from it. Uncle Bill's experience as a special needs teacher helped Mum in that brief time. This difficulty in feeding persisted for most of the first year. Luckily, I took a liking to Mum's lasagne, so she cooked a lot of it because it was one of the few things I would eat voluntarily.

Other challenges arose with returning home and managing my acquired disabilities. I remained scared of the dark because it was more difficult for me to maintain my balance. Bladder control was present only most of the time. Mum placed a bell next to my bed, so if I awoke during the night and needed to go to the toilet, I would ring the bell, and she would come to my aid. Thankfully she had always been a light sleeper.

At first, I could not stand in our shower, which was in the bath. The neurological damage I had suffered caused an uncontrolled tightening of my muscles, known as spasticity. This was due to disrupted signals to the brain and resulted in me being unable to squat or even bend my legs to the degree required to get up from or down to the ground. This meant I needed to be lowered into and lifted out of the bath. Again, Uncle Bill came to the rescue during his stay with us. Conscious of my 16-year-old modesty, Mum always ensured that I was covered with a towel. I would not be able to manage the bathing task on my own for another three months. Uncle Bill was a significant support in assisting Mum to care for me during his time with us. After a 10-day stay, it was time for Bill to go back to his wife and children and his work in Australia. Bill helped Mum plan for my return to school life and suggested that we come over to Australia for a few months before the start of the next school year, so I could attend the school where he taught children with disabilities. This would mean that instead of part-time rehab, I would get full-time rehab.

Mum continued to take me to physiotherapy, hydrotherapy, and speech therapy. Because of my multiple rehabilitation appointments and medical reviews, it became necessary for Mum to buy a car. She got a loan and bought our neighbours' little green Mini.

In hydrotherapy, I would swim around in circles because of the paralysis and weakness on my left side. I could not swim in a straight line no matter how hard I tried, so Mum engaged a swim coach. Within one month I could swim in a straight line. It took a lot of concentration, but I did it! Hydrotherapy consistently made a significant difference in my physical abilities, and although I did not enjoy it very much, the results were undeniable.

Mum had a meeting with the principal and special needs teacher of the high school I attended in Christchurch to develop a plan to slowly integrate me back into school. I would have to repeat my 6th form year at the start of 1988, but planning was underway to ensure that I could slowly build up my tolerance for attending school. They decided that I would begin by attending school for one lesson per week. The class they chose was Religious Studies. Oh, joy! I was not that excited about this. Religious Studies was not a class I had enjoyed before my accident and did not inspire me after. At least one thing had not changed! In hindsight, however, it was a good choice. It was not too academically demanding, and there was no homework. In this class, you listened more than took part, and the goal was to get me in an environment of my peers again and give them a chance to adjust to the new Nicole.

Through the Accident Compensation Corporation (ACC), the no-fault insurance system in New

Zealand, my rehabilitation interventions in hospital and post-discharge were covered financially. This is significant for brain injury because at the time, the consensus was that the maximal recovery period for brain injuries was the first two years after injury. If I had not been supported in this way, I would not have had access to many of the interventions that I was privileged to receive because we could not have afforded them. Another intervention being trialled at the time was the use of computers to help with concentration. My memory and concentration were extremely poor, as evidenced by the fact that there were notes everywhere in our house: on the front door, my mirror, the fridge. I struggled to remember what I had done yesterday, and my forgetfulness compromised my ability to plan.

I began a computer course that was funded by the ACC. The course was held at Ferrymead in Christchurch. It was a small class aimed at improving memory and concentration skills whilst learning to use a computer. Computers were still new at that time. We did not yet have them in classrooms at school. In fact, at school, there were a few electronic typewriters, but we still mostly had manual typewriters to learn to type on. I attended the course for a few hours, a few days per week.

KEY LEARNINGS
- Small steps are essential to achieving improvements in the early stages after a brain injury.

- The brain-injured person may require guidance in the form of boundaries to manage fatigue with activities. In those early days, I could not cognitively recognise when I was tired and had a propensity for just pushing myself, which could be both dangerous and counterproductive, as I would make more mistakes when tired and would also be more clumsy and more likely to fall over.

- Fatigue is likely to be significant and may remain a long-term issue. Breaking tasks up into small chunks is one strategy that was often used in my rehabilitation pathway, from the one hour, two days per week of being in a classroom with my high school peers to the very part-time computer course.

- Computer tasks were a great aid in helping to improve my memory and concentration, and now there are so many amazing memory challenge computer games. Introducing some structure to computer-related activities may be helpful to assess improvements. For example, commencing with small steps, such as 10 minutes a day (with a timer) and increasing time as concentration improves.

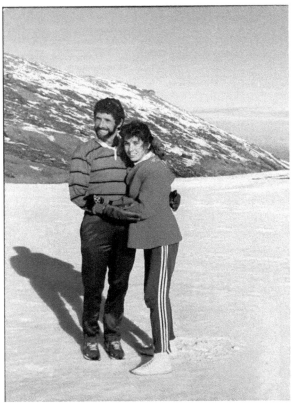

Uncle Bill and Nicole at Mt Cook, 1987

Chapter 7

Rehabilitation in Australia

After consultation with my practitioners, we decided that it would be beneficial to go to Australia for more active rehabilitation, to spend time with family, and to have a well-deserved holiday. At the end of the school term, we left for Australia. I was excited to be going.

My memory was nothing short of terrible. The heavy medication I was on to prevent seizures did not help my memory and concentration, but it was a necessary evil. I was not sure what to expect in Uncle Bill's class at the special needs school in New Farm, Brisbane. We were staying in Brisbane at the home of Uncle Jim, my mother's twin brother. I lacked a lot of insight into my appearance and behaviours and did not consciously identify as a person with a disability, nor did I want to. I was a little reluctant to be included in a special needs class, but Uncle Bill framed it as a role where I would be his assistant, so I went along with it, albeit reluctantly.

Working with people with disabilities spans three generations in my family. My grandfather used to do volunteer work one day per month at Montrose, an institution for people with disabilities. He was a hairdresser and would do free haircuts on that day. Before my accident, I had taken part in some volunteer experiences through my high school that involved working with people with disabilities, so being around kids with disabilities was not foreign. I would be at the school only one day per week for the first few weeks.

Bill picked me up that first morning to take me to school, and I was very nervous. I had no idea what to expect, how I would relate to the other children, or how they would relate to me. Bill introduced me to the other children, one by one. There were around nine kids in the class. The day was very interactive, and the first exercise was learning to throw and catch a ball. It was a small beach ball, very soft, and easier to manage for kids with dexterity issues. I had fun working with the kids to practise this skill, and then there was storytelling, reading, and singing songs.

I ended up enjoying my time at the school, and I have fond memories of the children. I remember a young man named Clive. He had limited verbal skills and was in a wheelchair, but he was Mr Personality and had a smile that lit up a room.

When the school holidays in Australia began, we went over to Uncle Bill's holiday house on Stradbroke Island. It was a lovely time, with sunshine, sand, and ocean waves crashing around us. The next part of our holiday was a trip up to Magnetic Island, where my Uncle Geoff had a house.

My childhood friend Duane joined us at Magnetic Island. Mum and Duane's mum, Mavis, used to work together at Wilfred Owen, a cosmetics and toiletries factory in Christchurch. Duane was also an only child, and we used to play together as kids. Duane had sometimes joined us on holidays over the years. He had visited me regularly in the hospital.

Staying at Uncle Geoff's house was quite the novelty for us. My Uncle Jim described it as like staying in Taronga Park Zoo! The house was set in bushland, and although it had walls and a roof, there were no actual doors or windows. We developed a verbal system for privacy when we went to the toilet or had a shower because there was no door! Our verbal cue was to shout, 'Flag Up' or 'Flag Down'!' As I said, it was quite the novelty!

In the morning, you could hear birds chirping as well as rustling in the trees from the many animal species. We were told there were no buses into the principal centre of Magnetic Island, so when we wanted to go into town, we had to walk a few kilometres. I was still a little unsteady on my feet and continuing to gain strength, so this was a challenge, but it was also good practise for balance and endurance.

After our holiday on Magnetic Island, we returned to Brisbane. Soon it would be time to return to New Zealand and repeat my 6th form year.

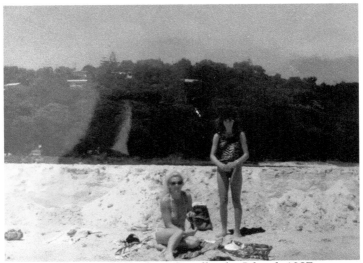

Mum and Nicole at Stradbroke Island, 1987

Chapter 8

Return to an Altered Reality

Upon returning to our home in Christchurch, Mum once again met with my school principal and the special needs teacher. Although I had made some good improvements whilst in Australia, they decided that I would continue with a reduced course load of four subjects instead of five. My classes would be with the students who had previously been in the year behind me, but I would still have access to the Form 7 common room where my previous classmates would hang out on breaks, etc.

Mum started back at Polytech to finish her Registered Nurse degree, and we attempted to navigate life with an altered reality.

It had now been eight months since I had sustained a severe head injury, and I was reassessed by the neuropsychologist. I had last been assessed at four months postinjury, and the neuropsychologist had described me as 'disinhibited, giggly and insightless'. He undertook various memory, intellectual and, visuospatial ability assessments, and the results included:

- Information processing and non-verbal memory remains significantly impaired.
- Scores on word fluency are impaired.
- Mood is much more appropriate with no sign

of the frank disinhibition evident four months postinjury.

- Recall of stories is unchanged, remaining low average but with no sign of confabulation or automatic speech.
- New verbal learning is in the average range.
- Immediate recall of non-verbal material is now average, though delayed recall remains significantly impaired.
- Visuospatial ability is impaired.

My teachers noticed that I was a different student from the pre-accident Nicole. I was attentive and quiet, trying to absorb the information being taught to me. I could no longer get away with not paying attention. I was also in classes with people I did not know, which reduced my confidence in being openly verbal. Memory issues were obvious just from a visit to our house. Trying to remember things was a daily challenge.

Prior to the accident, I had been at the top of my class in Teeline–a shorthand style. Upon returning to school in 1988, I chose Teeline as one of my four classes, but I literally had to learn this shorthand language from scratch again. I presumed it would be easier for my brain to relearn this information since I had been so adept at it before my injury. With a lot more work and focus, I was keen to maintain my 'first in class' status. So many things about myself had changed on 19 June 1987 and would never be the same, but I hoped my accomplishments in Teeline would be unchanged.

At the end of the school year, they awarded me a certificate for being 'first in class' for Teeline. I did not do so well in my other subjects, despite a concerted and genuine effort. I failed English, even though it had been one of my better subjects pre-injury and I had received extra tutoring. In addition to that, I even used a tape recorder to record the English lessons, so I could listen after class for memory reinforcement!

The return to school brought more glaring realities to light. I was different, although much of the impact to my brain was not immediately obvious. I attended a very supportive school that made every resource they had available to enable me to return. I now walked with a limp, smiled crookedly due to facial paralysis, and was uncoordinated. My physical education teacher tried to encourage me to return to netball, but I was so afraid of the comparison of my performance before and after the accident that I just ignored the offer. My medical team had strongly advised me not to engage in any contact sport due to the risk of re-injuring my brain, so returning to hockey was out of the question. I was no longer the carefree teenager with a rebellious spirit that my high school friends had once known. I was now somewhat of a responsibility because I wasn't able to be independent, and I could not do many of the things other teenagers were experimenting with at that age. I was so vulnerable. Many of my pre-accident friends distanced themselves from me. I do not blame them. They were young, and it was more important to be cool and to be seen to be cool. My behaviour was still challenging. I could not understand how difficult my accident and its consequences were for them because I was not walking in their shoes, but this poem, written by my high school friend Sara, provides some insight:

8pm they say it happened.
Hit and run it was.
What made him leave you
by yourself,
is something only he will know

It scared us all you know.
You read about it all the time,
but never think
it will happen to someone you know

It's changed us all,
some way or another – little or big.
You realise how precious friendship really s,
and not to see people for what they may try to
be,
but instead to see them as they are inside

The first few days
Were the worst of the lot.
Not really knowing what you were going to do.
We went to church on the Sunday night,
and prayed that very soon you'd be alright

So to see you
improving day by day,
is quite unexplainable.
To see your response to what we say,

> *to sit there cracking jokes,*
> *is just a great delight*
> *to all of us around*

> *So we know and pray,*
> *that you'll come through,*
> *shining all the way*

My young, brain-damaged mind did not understand at the time why my friends needed to distance from me, and I became depressed. On top of adjusting to disability issues, the epilepsy medication seemed to delay any significant recovery in memory and concentration and contributed to my depression. My brain injury had also exposed the traumas I had buried beneath the proverbial carpet, and I grieved for my father as if he had just died. Other traumas from childhood, such as sexual abuse, also came to the surface, and this was another reason for my spiral into a deep depression.

Mum could see that I was depressed, but I would not talk about it. I become more introverted. Mum shared her concerns with our local GP, but he had no answers because whenever he asked me how I was, I said that I was wonderful. I was always smiling in front of other people. Mum sensed that I was at risk for self-harm, and in desperation, she went through my room, searching for any clues to reinforce her intuition. I had been writing poetry, suicidal poetry, and she found the scrunched-up paper containing my depressed words regarding my experience with the head injury in my rubbish bin.

LIVING-DEAD

We could be called the living dead,
Surrounded by a wall of complete nothingness,
and therefore, it is many tears that are shed

We all share a common problem in the end,
one of devastation and loneliness,
and we can't be sure if that will mend

There is a newfound isolation to face.
Some refuse this,
therefore, they leave this world without a trace

We do have the knowledge up there,
but it is locked inside.
However, it is something we desperately want
to share.
The frustration of getting people to understand,
listen and care,
to comprehend the little, we have to share

It takes a while longer and more pain to learn,
just to unlock what is trapped inside,
and as we wait, we burn

So, to the people that do not want to learn to
comprehend
I ask YOU
Where do we turn in the end???

Nicole Yeates, August 1988

Prior to the accident, I could not have written
poetry to save my life. When a school homework

task required any kind of poetry, I would beg Mum to write it for me. My brain injury seemed to unlock a previously hidden talent, and I was now writing poetry that came straight from my heart and showed my emotional pain. She took the poetry to our GP, Dr McCormack, and he immediately referred me to a clinical psychologist, Dr Richard Wheeler.

I continued writing private poetry to express my pain.

HELL

This place is like hell.
I want them to listen,
but I am trapped in this shell,
and there is no way out.
In the shade with no sense of life,
or what it is meant to be.
Life, the word that is Godforsaken,
but to be brought into it,
I was so mistaken.

Nicole Yeates, 1988

Dr Wheeler was literally a lifesaver! He used cognitive behavioural therapy, in addition to visualisation and meditation techniques, to restore my psychological well-being. We actively worked on visualisation techniques to heal my brain, including my epilepsy. I would visualise my brain as a bunch of tangled spaghetti or rope or whatever my preferred visual was on the day, and under guided meditation, I would slowly put those mangled pieces back together in an ordered pattern. I also practised this technique at home, with a meditation tape Dr Wheeler had given me. I so wanted to be able to drive a car one day, but I needed to be seizure-free and get medical approval. It was a big goal.

Because of the resurfacing of the sexual abuse inflicted on me as a seven-year-old, and which I had kept secret for <u>seven years</u>, I became withdrawn again and could not tolerate being touched affectionately. My abuser had threatened to kill my mother if I told anyone, so the secret had remained within me until my mother was reviewing a book with me, which explained sexuality, when I was 14 years of age. I had not really fathomed what had happened to me until it was explained thru this book. I started to cry, and my mother asked why I was crying. I then told her of the sexual assault by a friend of our neighbours. Mum reported it to the police in Christchurch, but we did not hear any more. Mum did not know his proper name or where he lived. Our neighbours did not believe the accusation and would not give us his details to give to the police. My brain injury blew the lid off these memories, and Dr Wheeler recommended that I begin massage therapy to address my inability to respond emotionally or physically to touch. Besides my childhood trauma, a brain injury itself can cause a loss of emotion:

'Emotion dysregulation is a common
phenomenon after brain injury, often

*compromising socio-emotional adjustment and
participation. There has been little research
exploring the mechanisms by which brain
damage impacts emotion regulation'* (Salas,
2013).

The unpacking of so many buried emotions resulted in heightened disconnectedness. That disconnectedness can still be present to this day, to a lesser degree, and can present as a lack of empathy. For Mum, my lack of emotion was initially one of the hardest things to accept. I could not even receive a hug or affectionate touch. If she tried to cuddle me, I would stiffen and turn cold. ACC funded a course of massage therapy after some advocacy by Mum, and I began treatment with a massage therapist named Miggs.

It was about a year after my accident that the realisation set in for Mum: her baby girl who left on 19 June 1987 was not coming back, ever. She initially had held out hope that as I got back to 'normal' routines, I would become my old self. That was not to be, and it took about a year for Mum to accept that on some level. She was devastated for both of us. Mum recalls me telling Dr McCormack at an appointment one day that the old Nicole was gone and stating, 'I am not Nicole anymore. I am Simone.'

This was heartbreaking stuff for a mother to hear. She needed some time away to reflect, accept, and build strength. Although Mum needed to get away, she was not yet confident enough to leave me on my own in the house. My friend Nena agreed to stay with me during the school holidays while Mum went to a silent spiritual retreat at the nuns' residence in central Christchurch. It was a 10-day retreat that Mum found very healing, and it gave her hope for the future. She worked through the anger associated with the man who had hit me, the loss of the child she once knew, and the death of my father. She was now ready to face the continued challenges.

Remember the promise/bribe that was made to try to wake me from the coma? Mum stayed true to her promise and bought me a puppy dog. I named him Timothy, after the young man who had shared my journey but was not fortunate enough to survive his battle. Little Timothy was a black and white collie who brought me great joy and was a wonderful companion. We walked along the beach daily with Timothy.

I wanted to get back to some of the activities I had been involved in before my accident, so I tried to return to babysitting later in 1988. I may have looked like the former Nicole, but I was not, and the return to babysitting did not last long. I forgot to turn up for jobs and could not be relied upon. The parents stopped asking me to work after a few of these incidents. To help with my concentration and memory, Mum arranged for me to work on Saturday mornings at a library in Christchurch. It was the library at Polytech where she was getting her nursing degree. Mum would drop me off and then pick me up two hours later. My role involved sorting books in alphabetical order on the shelves. I do not think I particularly enjoyed the work, but it was a good start for helping my brain with problem-solving tasks. Somewhere around this time, Andrew, the man I had learned to walk with in hospital, also came back into my life.

Mum had been seeking support from the Brain Injury Association in Christchurch, and Andrew had attended one of their regular monthly meetings. I was still trying to be 'normal' and hung on to my denial of my disabilities as much as I could. I would not go to the brain injury support groups. Andrew approached Mum at one meeting and mentioned that he remembered me and would like to see me again. We met again in June 1988, and we would end up dating for nearly a year. Andrew was two years older than me, and Mum was less than thrilled about our relationship, but I had a lot of fun with him. In my last year of school, 1989, Andrew introduced me to nightclubbing, dancing, and pushing boundaries again.

I was becoming more independent now, and I craved even greater independence. To get my driver's licence, I needed to be seizure-free for 12 months and get medical approval to drive. The neurological report dated 15 April 1988, recommended that I be three years seizure-free before ceasing anti-convulsant medication. At this point, my last seizure had been a focal fit during October 1987. I was beginning to think about my future and leaned towards more administrative subjects at school. With support from Mum and Miggs, I was offered a part-time role after school two days per week to go into the Massage Centre's office and do some filing. Sorting files in alphabetical order was great for helping improve my memory and concentration, and I enjoyed the feeling of accomplishment in completing these tasks. It was a different environment than the library where I didn't really have the opportunity to talk to people. The office staff at the Massage Centre were lovely, and this small activity helped boost my confidence in social and work-related activities.

KEY LEARNINGS

- If you have experienced a brain injury and are a student of any sort, I highly recommend that you contact your school's disability support person to help you to increase your likelihood of success with your studies. This can involve extra tutorial time, reduced study load, approval for extra time to complete assignments, etc.

- If you are returning to work, you could receive assistance from a brain injury support service or occupational rehabilitation provider to help you negotiate flexible work arrangements with your employer.

- If your injury barriers are preventing a return to work, I recommend that you consult with an occupational rehabilitation specialist, such as an occupational therapist or rehabilitation counsellor. They may assist with pathways that will help you increase your work capacity. This may involve a vocational assessment to identify your key strengths, work experience, and interests concerning suitable employment.

- A vocational specialist may also be able to suggest some suitable volunteer work to build your tolerance for work-related duties.

- Our brains cannot tell the difference between real and made-up imagery. It is why we can cry at a scene in a movie. Our unconscious minds do not understand that the person who just died in the movie is not real. You can create your own movie about yourself by imagining you in the best light. Imagine your brain healing.

- Denial of disability can be a double-edged sword. It can drive you, but it can harm you too. Behaviours that move you away from your desired outcome can be driven by denial. For example, I wanted to be like my teenage friends and experiment with alcohol. By doing that, I could feel more normal, like part of the group, but I would have been moving further away from my goal because I would have been doing my brain harm. I didn't want to be part of a support group because of my denial, but by participating, I would have learned so much more about what strategies, tools, and treatments have worked for other people.

Chapter 9

Final Year of High School and Further Study

In January 1989, my neuropsychologist wrote to my GP, advising that I had remained seizure-free, despite the subtherapeutic level of phenytoin I was taking for epilepsy. He recommended reducing my dosage sequentially over six weeks, followed by further neurological review in six months. I had been working with Dr Richard Wheeler for around nine months by this time, and I was on track to be medication-free for epilepsy ahead of the predicted three-year time frame.

For my last school year, I chose subjects based more around my interests than academics and continued with just four subjects. For example, there were Art History classes in the boys' high school across the road from us. My interest was not in Art History but in the boys! My new high school friend Erin and I enrolled in the class. During classes, we rated those boys in every category imaginable and sent out invitations for parties at Erin's house. We had fun in that class!

Finishing high school had been a long-term goal of mine from the age of five. After my first day of primary school, I proudly came home and announced to Mum, 'I am going to go to school right to the very end!' My accident had given this goal more importance. Telling me I could not do something was akin to waving a red flag in front of a bull!

My poor memory and organisational skills were sometimes very embarrassing. I cannot remember how many times I had to go to the administration office and ask for tampons because I would forget to bring them to school with me! I felt humiliated by my inability to remember, but the ladies at the front office were friendly and non-judgemental. My menstrual cycle did not return for 18 months postinjury because of the stress on my body.

My final neurological assessment to determine permanent incapacity payment was on 19 May 1989, just shy of two years post-accident. The neuropsychologist stated:

> 'Her overall performance on WAIS-R was today in the low average range, which is significantly below likely pre-morbid functioning.'

> 'She has set herself the goal of a 7th form certificate, this being a prerequisite for a beautician course in Australia. It is likely that Nicole would have significant difficulty in seeing through these two consecutive goals.'

> 'In the early stages of her recovery, Nicole was markedly disinhibited, and indeed her demeanour is still a little euphoric and at times facile. Nicole's problem-solving skills have

undoubtedly been compromised, such that she would benefit from working in structured and closely supervised situations. I feel sure that Nicole will get back to some form of work, but I fear that it may not be as easily achieved as she currently imagines.'

Perhaps I was a little 'euphoric and facile', but I needed to prove those doctors wrong! This became a driving motivation for many years.

They also cleared me to try for my driver's licence. On 9 June 1989, my neurosurgeon provided a letter addressed to the Ministry of Transport, confirming that I was medically fit to drive. I failed the first practical driving test, but I passed the second time.

I had decided to pursue a career in beauty therapy, and this required that I finish high school. I also needed to improve my grade in mathematics and get a biology qualification to increase my chances of being accepted into the private beauty therapy college in Australia that I wanted to attend. The year 1989 was really the catalyst for improving my social skills more than anything. I had accepted the fact I would not be going to university and selected a career pathway I thought was more achievable. My interest in psychology remained, and during my last semester of high school, I also took a psychology course at night school. Some of the most helpful information I learned in this course was about memory aids and tricks, and I put these strategies to work.

The end of school came quickly. It had been a busy year: making new friends, exploring my relationship with Andrew, discovering my abilities further, and understanding some of my limitations. Ever the independent young woman at heart, I decided I would drive to Queenstown (about six hours south of Christchurch) and explore the world on my own. I even wrote a poem about this:

The joy of being able to be totally me,
the feeling of a real person, being free.
No strings of attachment, no wires,
doing whatever my heart desires.
Being able to use my restricted mentality,
as dreams turn into eventual reality,
I begin to find absolute fidelity.
I learn to grow, I learn to exist,
the feeling of freedom, I cannot resist.

The day after I finished high school, I moved to Queenstown. Mum and I had previously lived in Queenstown for four years, and I still had some friends down there. I booked into a camping ground that was owned by Mum's former employer, and through networks there I heard about a job vacancy at a small restaurant in the Queenstown Mall. I went down to the restaurant and asked if the job was still available, and they hired me to work that night. I had no experience, but they did not seem to mind. I can laugh now, but I was the worst waitress ever! I could not remember who ordered what and mucked up plenty of orders. The employer never asked me to work again. I was receiving fortnightly incapacity payments from ACC, which was enough to get by, but I had been working for many years of my young life already, and I wanted to continue. It was a way that I could feel a sense of normalcy. My networking skills were better than they had been pre-accident because I was more outgoing now. Through networking, I gained some work cleaning motel rooms. I also worked at an upmarket restaurant as a kitchen hand. The chef at the restaurant was looking for an extra flatmate, so I moved out of the camping ground and into a unit with him and two other young ladies. I am still friends with one of those flatmates after all these years!

I did not receive any career counselling throughout my rehabilitation, and my decision to pursue a career in beauty therapy was one that I came to independently and with Mum's support. Mum had always taught me to take pride in my appearance, and during the holidays after my return to school, she sent me to a modelling/deportment school. During this course, I learned how to do my makeup and walk on a catwalk (even though I still walked with a limp). The cost of the beauty therapy diploma I wanted was over $6,000 in New Zealand, but in Australia, it was just over $3,000. The assessment of my permanent impairment was determined, and I was paid $21,000 for my permanent injuries. My application to attend beauty therapy college was accepted, and Mum and I packed up and moved to Australia. I paid for the course from my compensation payout.

Mum sold our duplex in New Brighton, and we moved to Australia on 20 January 1991. I began a full-time beauty therapy course at Bellevue Beauty Academy the next day. Mum started her post graduate nursing training in Australia.

I remained determined to 'prove the doctors wrong', and my attitude was, 'I will gain meaningful work!' I wanted more out of life than the predictors based on anatomy and physiology. I studied hard for my beauty therapy diploma and developed memory retention skills, using much of the information from my psychology course. This involved mnemonics and stimulation of the memory through repetition, rote learning, and utilising different senses, e.g. for anatomy and physiology classes, I would draw the different muscles and visualise them. I graduated from the program during December 1991 and began my first full-time job as a beauty therapist during February 1992 at Zorbas Hair & Beauty in Carindale, Brisbane.

KEY LEARNINGS

- Visualisation and meditation were important factors in my recovery, and a psychologist or meditation specialist may help you find a system that will work for you.

- Although career counselling was not available to me when I was deciding about my future working life, there are now several different avenues you can access to discover suitable employment options. Speaking with a career counsellor or rehabilitation counsellor who specialises in working with people with disabilities may help you find and pursue work you will enjoy, taking into consideration both your limitations and your strengths.

- Taking small steps towards larger goals is essential.

Chapter 10

My Accident, the 'Gift' That Keeps on Giving. More Change Ahead

I did not realise the impact that working on my feet all day would have. As a result of the malfunction of my feet, due to developing 'foot drop' whilst in a coma, I had developed claw toes. This is due to a neurological response to brain trauma when ligaments and tendons have tightened to cause the toe's joints to curl downwards. This meant that when I wore closed-in shoes, I would get painful bunions on the tops of my toes. Enclosed shoes were required in the salon environment, and my ankles would swell because of being on my feet all day. My feet were painful, and after five years in the beauty industry, it became obvious that I would need to change careers due to these issues. I wore orthotics in my shoes to help with the drop foot and ankle swelling, and I researched alternative work. I now had some management experience, having managed other people's salons in my time as a beauty therapist, so I decided to study business management. I got my diploma in business management and initially got a job as an administrative assistant with a national media company.

Whilst studying for my diploma, I met my future husband, Michael. Around the time I met Michael, I also consulted an orthopaedic surgeon regarding my feet. He examined my claw toes and recommended surgery to straighten them. The surgery was successful, and after four weeks with both feet in plaster casts, I had straight toes and could wear enclosed shoes again without pain. Michael and I bought a house on Bribie Island. I had many experiences with him that I had never dreamed of before, including moving to Bowen and picking tomatoes for work and working in a sawmill, grading and lugging timber! None of this was what I had aspired to, but it helped keep food on the table and a roof over our heads. Michael was and is a good person. Our backgrounds were just too different, and our marriage would only last for two years before I left. During our marriage, we tried to have children but without success. I thought it was because of his excessive marijuana smoking and heavy drinking, but after our marriage ended, he soon got some other woman pregnant. I would not learn this until about 12 years later, for when I left the marriage, we did not speak again until Facebook happened. He also did not know that I had been diagnosed with stage IV endometriosis about four years after our marriage ended, so the probability of us ever having children was extremely low.

Because of the success of the surgery to straighten my toes, I ended up going back to beauty therapy and salon management. I was 29 years old by this time, and I was thinking of the years ahead, my career, and my achievements. Being able to retire comfortably on beauty therapist wages did not seem likely. My interest in psychology had not faded over the years, and given the stepping stones in my career that I had already achieved, I pondered the possibility of university. My achievements to date showed that I did not need to work in a supervised environment, as the neuropsychologist had predicted. I had successfully completed more than one qualification by this stage, and I wanted to retire one day on more than the minimum wage. As a beauty therapist, the most I ever earned was $30,000 in a year. It would take another couple of years, some encouragement from my friend David and significant research into different careers I could navigate within the disability or psychology sectors. I seemed to have an instinct for rehabilitation counselling, as even before I knew anything about it, I was contacting employers to do informational interviewing to learn more about the career path of a rehabilitation counsellor. Informational interviewing would end up being a technique they would teach me at university! One of the companies I contacted was CRS Australia. I wanted to know how much rehabilitation counsellors earned, the potential for career progression, and what the best and worst things about the work were. Once I had all this information, I applied for university. As I was mature in age and had not completed my early schooling in Australia, I had to sit a pre-entry exam on math, science, and English. English and science I was reasonably comfortable with, but mathematics had never been my strong suit. It was, however, one of Mum's strengths, so she tutored me in all the basics I had missed at school.

My preferences for university were psychology and rehabilitation counselling. Given that I had no academic track record, I knew that psychology would be a stretch, but if you do not try, you do not know. My friend David got the results before I did. He was the one who told me that I had been accepted into the rehabilitation counselling program at Griffith University. I was ecstatic and nervous. Some doubts tried to creep into my consciousness, but I wanted to give university my best shot! The rehabilitation counselling degree was a three-year, full-time program. For me, it was double full-time, as I needed to work to fund my studies.

Being a very independent person, I refused Mum's offer to move back home to reduce expenses while I completed the program. However, during the first semester, my landlord notified me of a rent increase, and I could no longer realistically make it work financially. I had scored a part-time job managing a small beauty salon, and even with Austudy, it was not a lot of money. About halfway through the first semester, I moved back home with Mum. I studied hard using all the same memory strategies that I had used in my previous studies, but I also tape-recorded lectures and listened to them, typed them, read them, and reread them. I created tests for myself and researched, researched, researched. . . . I worked hard at retaining information.

Towards the end of the first semester (2003), I experienced constant bleeding and terrible period pain. After some tests and scans, they diagnosed me with polycystic ovarian disease, and I required surgery. This would be the first of many surgeries. During surgery, the medical team discovered stage IV endometriosis. It was no wonder I had so much pain–the endometriosis had moved my organs to places they should not have been. An oncology surgeon was requested to assist with separating my ovary from my bowel and putting my organs back in place. During the surgery, my bowel was perforated, and they signalled the emergency bell. Once again Mum would be left in a hospital waiting room, knowing that the emergency was because of me but powerless to do anything about it. Despite my being a public patient, they transferred me to a private room to recover, and they administered a plethora of antibiotics. Bowel perforation is a critical situation. To allow my body to heal, they gave my reproductive system a break for six months via a medication called Zoladex. The specialist was surprised that I had not experienced any period pain until recently because the endometriosis was significant and severe. This was my second indication of residual paralysis remaining in my body. The first had occurred about a year earlier when I was working in a beauty salon in Brisbane, and the salon owner offered to do some cosmetic eyeliner tattooing for my birthday. As the needles penetrated around my right eye, I could feel every prick, and it was not pleasant. The right eye took about 90 minutes because I was blinking so much. When she went to my left eye, I could not feel as much sensation; therefore, I did not blink as much, and it only took about 45 minutes to do the left eye. I knew I had a remarkably high pain tolerance, but I did not fully understand why. Through future medical mishaps, I would learn how dangerous this high pain tolerance could become.

The Zoladex medication put my body in temporary menopause with all of its side effects–hot flashes, sleepless nights, moodiness, poor concentration, and memory issues (on top of already compromised concentration and memory). The return to university post-surgery was tough. If someone sneezed during class while I was reading, I would need to start the sentence again. This was going to be a problem for exams, so I contacted the disability counsellor at the university, and at her request, I got a letter from my gynaecologist outlining the side effects of Zoladex and the extra supports needed because of its impact on my brain injury. Thankfully, they arranged for me to sit my first semester final exams in a room alone with one exam supervisor. At the end of the semester, I ended up with one Pass and three credits. I was on my way, and my grades continued to improve from there!

I continued to work in beauty therapy for up to 20 hours per week during those first two years of university, but in my last year, I decided it was time to step out of my comfort zone and get some hands-on experience in the work I would do after graduation. I applied for a job doing personal care in a lady's home in the suburb neighbouring where I lived. I began to work for Marg, who was in her 50s at the time. She had severe cerebral palsy from a brain aneurysm soon after birth. Marg had a strong and feisty personality and did not let her disability become the barrier that many others in her circumstance might have. Despite relying on a roster of staff like me to handle all of her personal care, housework, feeding, etc., she worked full-time in disability research and owned her own home. She had a degree and had travelled overseas. Her sister rang each night to check on her, but Marg hired and fired her staff as she saw fit. Marg was inspiring!

KEY LEARNINGS

- Research into the suitability of job roles is critical to ensuring that you will be setting yourself up for success.

- Being proactive in disclosing your injury-related issues to the training institution upon enrolment will save red tape and wait times if you need the help.

Chapter 11

The Challenges of Work as a Rehabilitation Counsellor

In my last semester of university, I applied for work all over Australia. I did not really care where I went, so long as I had a job. I even applied to a Mt Isa mine! I ended up with two interviews in Coffs Harbour, New South Wales, a beautiful part of the world. I drove down there one weekend to attend the interviews, and I was successful in securing one of the positions. I had not technically finished university yet, as there was still one exam remaining. I found myself a cheap furnished unit to rent through an online search, packed my car one weekend in October 2005, and started my first job in Coffs Harbour in the occupational rehabilitation industry. A few weeks later, I went back to Brisbane to sit my ethics exam and ended up with an overall GPA of 5.5, which is in the credit range (a Pass is 4 and a High Distinction is 7). They offered me a spot in the honours degree program, but now I had had a taste of work and a decent income. There was no way I was going back to being a poor student! It was soon after moving to Coffs Harbour that I met the love of my life, Greg.

About six weeks after starting my new job and

learning all of their processes, a new computer database, and the New South Wales workers compensation legislation, I could no longer deny the fact that my memory was not holding up. I thought about new strategies I could use to aid my memory. There were clients to remember, and with each client, there was an injury to remember, individual limitations to consider, work capacity mandated by their treating medical professionals to recall when seeking work opportunities for them, legislation to remember, the company database to learn and so much more. My brain was overwhelmed by so much information, so I took a step back and went back to the basics of memory retention strategies. I created tables to record my individual clients' names, the details of their injury limitations, their agreed-upon job goals, and the interventions required to assist them in reaching those goals.

Client	Job Goal	Limitations/ Barriers and Work Capacity	Interventions required	Outcome/ Completion Date
A	Retail Assistant	10 kg lifting-capacity Fit for 15 hours per week Short term memory	Work hardening exercise program Development of memory strategies Develop compete-tive resume Cold canvass for suitable work trial opportunities Graduated Return to Work Program	Within 3 months

This helped, and I continued to use this table strategy, reviewing and updating it regularly to keep on track. Unfortunately, it had also become obvious to my manager that I was struggling. At my mid-probation review, my manager asked me how I thought I was doing. I was upfront and disclosed my injury, as I felt I was at risk of not making it through probation if they were not aware of why I was struggling. Such a disclosure could have worked against me, and I knew there was a risk, but despite forgetting things and being disorganised as a result, I had also been getting some fantastic results with clients, and I got along well with everyone in the workplace, so I was quietly hopeful. Thankfully, my manager could already see some improvement in my ability to cope with the work and was understanding and supportive because he appreciated the proactive strategies and independent problem-solving I had already put in place. There was no way I had worked this hard to come this far and not make it work! My manager was willing to keep me on, with more supervision.

I returned to Brisbane once again for my graduation, which was a very special day. Having achieved what I had worked so hard to obtain, I felt the need to write to the neurosurgeon and neuropsychologist to let them know that my 'facile and euphoric' self had indeed proved them wrong! I sent them a copy of my university transcript with a photo of myself in my graduation robe holding my degree and a pleasant letter thanking them for their good care of me and asking them to consider more than anatomy and physiology when making their future predictions. I explained my belief that a person's personality, support systems, belief systems, and willingness to work hard to reach personal goals also factor into outcomes. I received a response from the neurosurgeon, and he congratulated me on my achievement and advised that he also factors those things into his prognosis decisions. It was like a weight off my shoulders to receive this acknowledgement from a medical professional who had given us little hope of a positive outcome. I had not realised how much anger I had been holding on to because of those predictions, and I could now let it go.

I remained in my first role as a rehabilitation counsellor for 18 months and received some excellent mentoring. I am so glad I started my career in private practise. My confidence in my work increased because of the excellent results I was getting with placing injured workers into alternative employment. I applied for a role within government vocational rehabilitation, which involved a mixture of continuing to work with people on workers' compensation benefits but also job seekers within the Centrelink system receiving government-funded benefits, such as unemployment and disability payments. I was successful in winning this position with CRS Australia, and this job would involve my first foray into management within my occupational rehabilitation career. One year later, they promoted me to senior rehabilitation consultant (second in charge).

It was around this time that a friend and colleague, Kim, was getting married, and this led me to uncover a niche market in Coffs Harbour. Knowing I had a background in beauty therapy, Kim asked me to do her makeup for her wedding. I soon discovered there were plenty of mobile makeup artists in Coffs Harbour and plenty of mobile hairdressers, too, but no business provided both services under one roof. Instyle Wedding & Formal Services was born as a result. I started my hobby business in 2007 on weekends and initially hired two hairdressers. The business grew, and eventually, I had three contract hairdressers and two other contract makeup artists. The business became too big for me to manage on top of full-time work, so I ended up selling it to one of my contractors seven years later. My side business had become something of a lifeline for me along the way, though. Going to weddings on weekends was more fun than work for a long while, and this social connection would become more important than ever after losing Greg to bowel cancer.

The year from 2008 to 2009 was one of the hardest of my life. In 2008, Greg and I tried IVF to have children. The first IVF cycle was unsuccessful, and we decided to try a second time. It was an expensive and difficult process. The second lot of hormones caused cysts to grow on my ovaries at quite a rapid rate, and I had to have prompt surgery to remove them. Because of my complex endometriosis, my gynaecologist decided that I should have the surgery with a very experienced professor in Brisbane, and in November 2008 I travelled to Brisbane to undergo this surgery. Greg drove me up to Brisbane but had to return to work in Coffs Harbour. Mum was at the hospital with me, as she was living in Brisbane. After the surgery, Mum remembers that the surgeon appeared incredibly stressed, and he informed her that I had enough endometriosis for 10 women. He had removed a significant amount of the endometriosis along with the cysts. I was keen to get home and pushed for release. Upon returning to Mum's house in Brisbane, I was not feeling well but stayed quiet. My stomach was slowly expanding with what seemed like swelling, and I had no appetite. I tried to brush it off when Mum checked on me, but she could see I was extremely uncomfortable, and she checked my heart rate, which was high. Around 4:00 pm, Mum wanted to take me back to the hospital, but I said, 'Let's just see how I am in the morning.' Mum continued to check my heart rate, and at around 6:30 pm she called it. My heart rate had continued to increase even though I was sitting around doing nothing. Despite my protests, she called an ambulance. They transferred me to the Mater Hospital in South Brisbane, and at close to midnight, they called the theatre staff back to work, and I underwent emergency surgery. The surgeons found that I had a bowel perforation that was not detected during surgery, and I had become septic. The diagnosis was septicaemia. They had to remove a portion of my necrotic bowel, and they inserted an ileostomy bag on my stomach for my bowel motions. They placed me in an induced coma on life support following surgery, and despite feeling unwell himself, Greg began the road trip back to Brisbane from Coffs Harbour. He, too, was experiencing stomach pains but thought it was the stress of everything happening with me. I recovered from septicaemia and learned to live with a bowel bag, and I was discharged from hospital a few weeks later. Further surgery to remove the ileostomy bag occurred six months later.

Greg's stomach pains became worse, and on Boxing Day 2008, I ended up taking him to emergency. They provided him with some Movicol and sent him home with a referral for an ultrasound. A few days later, Greg had the ultrasound, and a request to undertake an MRI was made by the radiology staff at the same time. On New Year's Eve 2008, they diagnosed Greg with stage IV bowel cancer, and we began another fight for life. Greg had to have surgery to remove the tumour on his bowel, and the surgeon removed a tumour that weighed close to 2 kg. The doctor said that it was the biggest bowel tumour he had ever seen. It sadly explained why Greg could never lose the weight off his stomach. He was tall and slim but had a large belly, and despite us having a healthy diet and walking regularly, plus him playing golf regularly, the weight from his stomach would not budge. Now we knew why. Sadly, his battle with bowel cancer would be lost, and Greg died from pneumonia, secondary to bowel cancer, on 22 August 2009. I was heartbroken.

I threw myself into my work and my business and

just buried myself in things to do. This included training to be a mediator and doing postgraduate study in business-to-business marketing. A year later, I also took some time off to travel the world and explore life on my own, to reframe and figure out this life I now had to live without Greg.

KEY LEARNINGS

- Memory aids are an excellent resource when learning new tasks. I still use the table format to remind me of batches of information I need to remember whenever I start a new occupational rehabilitation role.

- Adding all time-dependent tasks into a calendar and setting reminders can be helpful.

- Positive injury disclosure–focus on strengths and solutions.

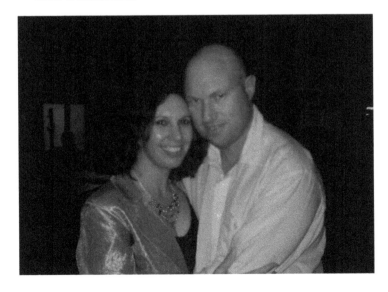

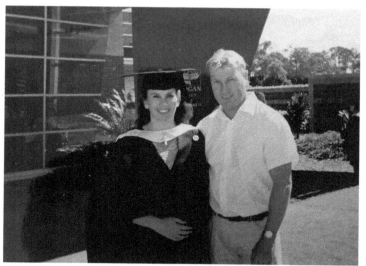

With Greg on Graduation day

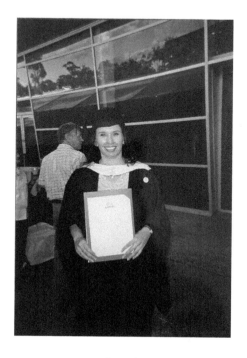

Chapter 12

Managing Life with a Brain Injury & Tools to Improve Your Life

I have been asked over the years whether I wish that the event that caused my brain injury had not happened. If I could go back and make a different decision the night of my accident, would I? It is a pointless question really, for we cannot change our past, we can only change our future–if we choose to. I chose to. Today, I continue to work in occupational rehabilitation as a rehabilitation counsellor and accredited mediator. I still love the work I do and enjoy the challenges and rewards of working with people who sometimes do not believe they can ever work again because of their injury limitations. My belief continues to be that everyone has strengths that they can use in some form. It does not have to be for formal work purposes. We all have knowledge and life experience that others can learn from; we have skills, talents, and knowledge that are individual to us.

Fatigue is still an issue for me, and my brain sometimes does not cooperate in letting me know that I am too tired to do cognitive tasks effectively.

Often it is not until I make obvious mistakes, my coordination becomes more compromised and I become clumsy, or other such incidents that I am 'made aware' that I should switch to less demanding tasks, or if time permits, have a rest. Rest can be challenging in the workplace, so if there are time-dependent, cognitive tasks I must complete, I will just double and triple proofread everything I have done. The key is to listen to the body's cues and take appropriate action.

A review of some online brain injury support groups will validate the fact that fatigue is common when recovering from a brain injury, and even for those with a good recovery outcome, fatigue can still be a challenge. Brain imaging research has found that injured brains work harder to perform at the same level as healthy brains (Johansson and Rönnbäck, 2014). After a brain injury, the brain's ability to function in an energy-efficient capacity is compromised, resulting in energy loss (Baycrest Centre for Geriatric Care, 2014). Fatigue is one of the most significant long-term challenges after a TBI.

Developing a positive mindset

Your current way of thinking may be keeping you where you are, but is that where you want to be? If you would like to improve your current situation, you likely need to start by changing your mindset.

- Developing a positive mindset (if you are not already manifesting this) will take a conscious effort. You may have heard about practising gratitude. This is a simple and reflective process you can add to your routine at the end of each day, to reflect on something positive that happened during your day. It may be as simple as receiving a friendly smile from a stranger or feeling gratitude for the comfortable roof over your head. Many studies have found that expressing gratitude increases optimism.

- There are numerous studies regarding the practice of meditation and how this regular practice can improve your mindset, improve your memory, help you manage stress more effectively as well as many other health benefits. Meditation is a form of brain training. There are multiple studies that show that meditation can actually change your brain. Of significance to people with a brain injury, is that there are even studies that show how meditation can increase the cortical thickness of the hippocampus. This is the area of the brain which oversees memory and learning! If you think meditation is boring, try reading 'Meditation as F*ck!', Master the Art of Meditation in 10 Days by Prof. Dr. Detlef Beeker. It is an easy read with 10 different easy to follow meditations you can do. Haven't got time? The quickest meditation he teaches is mini-meditation for 3 minutes!

- Try to surround yourself with positive people. When you seek out positive people, you will be influenced by solution-focused thinking and can-do attitudes. Being in such company can transform your own thinking. There are positive thinking groups that advertise for members such as personal development groups. Try googling 'positive thinking groups' in your area! Business networking groups are also often filled with positive, can-do thinkers. Groups such as Toastmasters teach people to be confident with public speaking. This can be a real challenge for a lot of people, but when you are surrounded by positive and supportive people, it is amazing how much more you can achieve.

- If you can join a gym or any type of exercise class, such as yoga, you can meet people trying to improve their lives, well-being, and fitness through exercise. Any group that focuses on personal development and growth is likely to include positive people. There is significant evidence that exercise is also good for the mind.

- Look for evidence in the stories of other people who have defied the odds. We cannot all achieve everything that someone else has, but we can all find inspiration to try something new.

- Learn to acknowledge and understand your strengths. We all have strengths we can build on. Understanding your strengths is a great way to increase your confidence. Seeking out pathways where your strengths can be utilised is an excellent way of building your new identity and increasing endurance. Participating in a transferable skills analysis with a vocational professional can help you identify these strengths and learn how they can be utilised within rehabilitation activities. For more information go to www.holdingontohope. com.au.

In the words of author Martin Seligman (2019),

> 'The key to learning optimism is learning how to recognise and then dispute unrealistic catastrophic thoughts.'

Do you believe that you are worthy of abundance in your life? We all have limiting beliefs that can hold us back from achieving our goals, but you can manifest abundance by changing your limiting beliefs. Pamela Millican-Hartnoll's poem on this subject sums it up beautifully:

LIMITLESS ABUNDANCE

I limit my abundance
And I really don't know why
I question if I'm worthy
When the chances pass me by

What if I let abundance in
You can have it all they claim
But I wanted things when I was small
And all that caused was pain

I have all these blocks to happiness
To success and wealth galore
I think, I should only have a little
Because its selfish to want more
But when I look around me
I see affluence everywhere
If I did allow the riches in
I know for sure I'd share

I wonder then if I can change
This odd idea I hold
That people like me can't have more
Or so it is, I'm told
Or maybe contemplate a way
To change my broken understanding
Let prosperity come rushing in
Faulty mindset notwithstanding

Release the wrong and false ideas
That abundance makes you bad
And clear the blocks to having more
Because to not to . . . would be mad

I think I should give it a try
It's here for all of us you see
My affluence takes naught from you
Nor does your wealth take from me.

Pam's affirmation for attracting abundance is *'Limitless abundance you are so welcome in my life'* (Millican-Hartnoll, 2020).

Ways to increase your motivation
- Experiencing setbacks or failures is disappointing, but you can use the lessons you have learned. Failing at something is ok because it doesn't mean you are a failure, it just means that something did not work out as you might have hoped. Failure can be temporary if you keep trying. As Thomas Edison stated, *'I have not failed 10,000 times–I've successfully found 10,000 ways that will not work'* (Fernandez, 2019).

- Plan small steps of success to get to a bigger goal. For example, if your goal is to return to work in some form, you might do a vocational preparation course (a statement of attainment or Certificate 1 or 2 level course) via a registered training organisation and gain some work experience after the course. You could participate in volunteer work to build up your tolerance for work. You could start a new hobby or interest to meet new people. There are lots of less demanding activities that could be trialled in pursuit of a larger goal. By completing these steps successfully, you will set yourself up for success in a workplace. If you are not able to reach your goal successfully, then utilising your gratitude practise will help you to realise the benefits you gained in trying.

'While bouncing back is a key part of the definition, resilient people are also good at learning from their mishaps and finding motivation in big or small adversities' (Hensch, 2016).

Ways to empower yourself within the medical model of treatment

- Research your treatment options and develop questions to ask your medical professionals.

- Join support groups to see what treatments have helped other people, and share your own tips too.

- Get involved in the decisions on what treatment is best for you by asking questions and getting a second opinion.

- Combine modalities (traditional and alternative/ natural), following review with your treatment team, of course. Complementary, natural alternatives are generally more accepted by the medical model of treatment.

- Treatment will need to continue outside of your formal treatment appointments if you are able. The more effort you put in, the more you will benefit. Continuing with your rehab on your own time may lead to faster results.

- Ask for your blood test results, scan results, and all other results. Keep copies of them and learn what they mean. This will help you ask valuable questions of your medical team and give you more power to be your own advocate.

I want to find suitable work, but should I disclose my brain injury to an employer?

Injury disclosure is a very personal decision, and I often review this with my clients prior to commencing the job-search process. First of all, the job goal you are aiming for needs to be suitable to maximise your chances of success. Does the job goal utilise some of your strengths? Are you able to complete the inherent requirements of the role? Inherent requirements are the essential requirements of the job. For example, if you are applying for a job as a truck driver, but you do not have a truck licence, the employer is under no obligation to hire you, whether you have a disability or not. You must be qualified for the job you are applying for. If you are qualified for the job, but your disability means that you may struggle with some aspects of it, the employer is required to make 'reasonable accommodations' to enable you to do the work. For countries who have anti-discrimination laws, the employer could be found to be discriminating if they do not hire you (or if they fire you) because of disability-related issues if it is found that job modifications, equipment, etc., could have been provided to enable you to do the work, and you can fulfil the inherent requirements of the work. In Australia and America, anti-discrimination laws do not require an employer to make adjustments or accommodations if the cost of doing so would be unreasonable. For example, if installing an elevator would be the only way to enable an employee with a disability to access areas of a worksite that were essential to the job, but the cost of providing the elevator was excessively high, it could be considered unreasonable to expect the employer to do this. Anti-discrimination laws may differ in each country, so it is important to know your rights.

It is also important to have medical approval from your specialist to confirm that you are medically fit to work. If the job you wish to undertake is safe, suitable, and sustainable, you will need to consider whether you want to disclose your injury or disability to the employer. Some people may choose to disclose during the application process. Some may choose to disclose during the interview process or after they get the job. Some may choose not to disclose at all.

Employers receive many applications for one vacant position, and I personally believe that the decision to interview someone following receipt of their application should be based on skills. If, however, you will need some significant (yet reasonable) work adjustments, they may take some time to implement, so advising the employer early on can build trust and facilitate a plan for your commencement. Approaching the discussion with a solution-focused framework will help your negotiations.

If the workplace modifications you require are less costly, such as an ergonomic chair, or are practical accommodations, such as adjusting work hours to cope with fatigue, it may be better to have those conversations at the interview, rather than in your application for the job.

If you have developed effective memory management strategies and other strategies to manage your injury limitations and have trialled your ability to cope with the work, you may not need to disclose your injury. This is a personal decision. If your injury is related to work insurance, however, you should talk to a lawyer regarding what you may be required by law to disclose on a job application form that seeks information about work-related injuries. This will differ between countries.

Strategies for managing and improving your memory
Brain injury can have a significant impact on your ability to remember, to plan, and to recall new

information or what happened yesterday. There are many different types of memory, but the main ones are categorised as long-term and short-term memory. You may be able to remember details of events from many years ago, such as learning how to multiply at school, or details of a holiday you had as a child. This would relate to your long-term memory. On the other hand, you may have difficulty recalling what you did yesterday, or you may struggle to recall the information you just read on the previous page. This is short-term memory.

A review of feedback in brain injury support groups shows that short-term memory issues are a frequent source of frustration and can lead to a person appearing disorganised and unreliable. The person may feel frustrated, exasperated, and disappointed with themselves when they forget things. Struggles with short-term memory can also cause embarrassment. The times I had to go to the administration staff at school to ask for tampons have definitely moved into my long-term memory because I was so embarrassed!

If you want the most from your memory, you need to give it the right nutrition and care. Are your actions moving you closer to your goal of a better memory or further away from the memory you want? In Norman Doidge's book *The Brain's Way of Healing* (2017), he writes about reducing the risks of dementia, and details the following evidence from a 2013 study:

"The breakthrough study was done by Dr. Peter

Elwood and a team from the Cochrane Institute of Primary Care and Public Health, Cardiff University, United Kingdom, and released in December 2013. For thirty years, these researchers followed 2,235 men living in Caerphilly, Wales, aged 45 to 59, and observed the impact of five activities on their health and on whether they developed dementia or cognitive decline, heart disease, cancer or early death. The Cardiff study was meticulous, examining the men at intervals over the thirty years, and if they showed signs of cognitive decline or dementia, they were sent for detailed clinical assessments of high quality. It overcame study design problems from eleven previous studies (discussed in the end notes).

Results showed that if the men did four or five of the following behaviours, their risk for cognitive (mental) decline and dementia (including Alzheimer's) fell by 60 percent:

- *Exercise (defined as vigorous exercise, or walking at least two miles a day, or biking ten miles a day). Exercise was the most powerful contributor to decreased risk of both general and cognitive decline and dementia.*

- *Healthy diet (as measured by eating at least three to four servings of fruits and vegetables every day).**

- *Normal weight (as measured by having a body mass index between 18 and 25).*

- *Low alcohol intake (alcohol is often a neurotoxin).*

- *No smoking (also a case of avoiding a toxin).*

*We know much more about diet and the brain since that study was initiated thirty years ago. For an up-to-date discussion on how diet, food sensitivities, glucose, insulin, and obesity affect brain health, and the relationship between exercise and insulin, see the neurologist David Perimutter's Grain Brain (New Your: Litt, brown, 2013)"

Many studies have proven that alcohol is neurotoxic, and this impacts the brain's neurotransmitters. Heavy drinking can also cause shrinkage in the hippocampus, the part of the brain that is associated with memory and reasoning. Over the years, and through my own study and practise with memory management techniques, I have found some tools that work for me and enable me to keep my life organised. To enable success with these strategies, it is important to minimise the distractions that can negatively impact your memory. Over the years, and through my own study and practise with memory management techniques, I have found some tools that work for me and enable me to keep my life organised. To enable success with these strategies, it is important to minimise the distractions that can negatively impact your memory. Where possible, I have found that the following guidelines are helpful to improve memory retention:

- If you are trying to do cognitive tasks such as reading a book, studying, writing a letter, etc., try to limit the distractions around you by finding a quiet place to focus.

- Take regular rest breaks to reduce fatigue.

Avoid starting cognitively demanding tasks if you are already tired.

- Carry a memory aid such as a memory app on your phone or a notepad with you all the time. Get into the habit of inputting or writing down your 'to-dos'.

- Try to focus on one task at a time, initially. Multitasking can be more challenging for the damaged brain. Try to be patient with yourself, as managing multiple tasks at a time may take some practise.

- Develop routines (like recording every appointment in your memory app and setting reminders).

- Learn strategies to improve your stress management. A psychologist or counsellor can help you. A stressed mind can become a more muddled mind, so limiting and managing stress is important.

Memory aids can become part of your life, and eventually, using the aids that work for you can become a positive habit and something you do automatically. It may take a couple of months to form this habit, but once you have mastered it, it will become a way of life, and you will not have to think about it. If you get used to using memory aids, your life will become more organised, and you can become less stressed and more independent. These bonuses are fantastic for helping to build confidence and self-esteem. Below you will find some of the memory aids that have worked for me.

Mnemonics

Mnemonics are a system or tool, developed to improve and assist our memory retention. There are many mnemonic methods that you can google. Mnemonics can be great for helping to remember lists. The ones I find easiest to use in everyday life are story mnemonics and acronyms to remember lists.

The story mnemonic is best utilised with outlandish stories, *and it can be fun too.* I use mnemonics if I am in a rush or do not have access to a resource to make notes. Just the other day, as I was walking out the door to do some errands, my mother asked me to get three grocery items on my way home. She asked me to purchase milk, tomatoes, and laundry detergent, so I made up a quick mnemonics story on my way to the car. I had lots of things to do in addition to getting the groceries, so it would have been a risk to rely on my memory without giving it some help. The following story helped me remember all the items when I arrived at the supermarket two hours later.

> *I was walking out the door when I slipped on a* **tomato** *and stained my pants, so I had to go back inside and use* **laundry detergent** *to remove the stain. As I waited for my pants to dry, I had a warm glass of* **milk** *to calm me down.*

When you use mnemonics, I recommend that you start with writing your normal shopping list, but leave off two to three items and use mnemonics to develop a story around them. You could turn this into a challenge for yourself, but while you are starting, it may be a good idea to have those missing items written on a separate piece of paper in your bag somewhere. It may take a couple of tries to get the hang of it.

You may remember acronym mnemonics from high school, when it may have been used to remember the periodic table in science class. You can use it to remember any list. Most of us know what a SIM card is, but how many can remember that it is the acronym for Subscriber Identity Module? Or perhaps you have heard of the acronym for treating a sprain, RICE?

Rest

Ice

Compress

Elevate

Acronyms are often easier to remember than their longer meanings. There are lots of ways you can use acronyms as memory aids.

Visuo-spatial awareness

If you have trouble putting do-it-yourself flatpacks of furniture or machinery together or find it difficult to navigate narrow spaces without bruising yourself, you may have issues with spatial awareness. This was an area of the psychological testing that I struggled with. Back in the '80s, as part of aptitude testing postinjury, I was given a picture and colour-coded blocks and was asked to create the picture with the blocks. I could not do it. As an adult, I started playing golf with Greg, but I could not hit the ball in a straight line, and then if I hit the ball too far, I couldn't find it, despite having perfect eyesight. I found the following techniques great for improving my visual-spatial awareness (and even my golf game!):

- Completing jigsaw puzzles. Start with easier ones and work your way up to the more complex ones.
- Visual-spatial brain training games.
- Playing chess.
- Playing bowls.

Today I continue to walk with a slight limp, which is not obvious to everyone. I continue to smile crookedly when I am tired due to the residual left-side paralysis in my face. I still have a very limited sense of smell, and I often forget words but remember the letter they start with. This is known as anomic aphasia. I still need to focus carefully when stepping onto elevator stairs or walking downstairs, but the most consistent challenge remains my memory and concentration. The strategies outlined above have become a natural part of my life now. People often comment positively on how organised I am! A client commented recently, 'God, you're sharp!' I had contacted him to remind him it was now the 60th day following his training and the last day he could go to the Safe Work NSW office to get his forklift licence. How did I remember? When the training company told me that they would provide him with a temporary licence, and he had 60 days to get the full licence, I added the date to my Outlook calendar!

I still very much enjoy my work in occupational rehabilitation, which brings me a great deal of satisfaction and reward. I have built a solid reputation as a rehabilitation consultant who helps injured people navigate complex psychological and physical barriers to work, resulting in a job outcome rate of up to 86% in a year for clients who need to move into different employment. This is something I am proud of. I have learnt a lot over time, not least of which is that I am NOT invincible, but I sure as hell am resilient, and I am confident that I have proven those doctors wrong!

My challenge for you
If you are tired of facing the challenges of life with impaired memory, I invite you to accept this memory challenge, with the goal of better memory management resulting in less frustration, more appointments attended on time, better management of bills, improved regularity of taking your prescribed medications, and increased confidence for organising your time and commitments. These are a few examples, but if you use the techniques described in this book, in liaison with the Holding On To Hope, RETIINK Memory app, I am confident you will be more than impressed with the results! Sound good?

Step 1: Complete the Memory Quizz. This will give a baseline to rate your progress over a 3-month period.

MEMORY QUIZZ

1. In the past three months have you received an overdue payment notice from any company you receive goods or services from? For example, your mobile phone provider
   □ YES □ NO

2. In the past three months, have you forgotten to attend more than one scheduled appointment or meeting? For example, a medical appointment or a meeting with a friend
   □ YES □ NO

3. In the past three months, have you ever forgotten to take your medication?
   □ YES □ NO □ Not Applicable

4. In the past three months, have you forgotten to complete the exercises or recommended actions prescribed by your treating professionals? e.g., complete home-based exercises, practice mindfulness or other activities to help your progress.
   □ YES □ NO

5. In the past three months, have you ever gone to a shop and forgotten something you intended to buy (such as a grocery item from the supermarket)?
   □ YES □ NO

6. Do your short-term memory issues cause you to feel frustrated?
   □ YES □ NO

7. Do you regularly forget to write down or add your 'to do' items to your calendar?
☐ YES   ☐ NO

Step 2. Set a date in your calendar for implementing a healthy diet and regular exercise into your lifestyle. Research 'brain injury diets' by talking to your health professionals or try googling it. Once you have decided on a date to implement your healthier diet and exercise regime, set a reminder for three months from that date, to do the quiz again.

Step 3: Follow the link below:

START IMPROVING YOUR MEMORY TODAY

Free Memory Cheat Sheet & Retiink Memory App Trial

Go to the following link

https://www.holdingontohope.com.au/memory-cheat-sheet

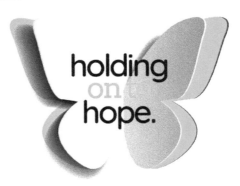

EPILOGUE

In the '80s, the medical consensus was that there was a two-year window for recovery from brain injury, and that was the end of progress. However, my brain was still improving more than 15 years postinjury, depending on the stimulus I was providing it. I made significant improvements during my university studies. Neuroplasticity is now well recognised, and there is more hope for better outcomes after a TBI. Am I fully recovered? No. The Nicole Yeates of 19 June 1987 died that night and will never return. I have had to accept a 'new me', but I am a fully functioning, very productive member of society who, despite a severe brain injury, has learned to (mostly) manage the effects. None of it is easy, there are no quick fixes, and it takes hard work, consistent effort, and small steps to make a pathway to improvement. I am using my experience to make a difference in the lives of others who suffer from injuries that change their lives, whether physical or psychological (and sometimes both), through my work in occupational rehabilitation. Maybe I am still facile and euphoric, but I am happy with myself. It took a lot of years to achieve that.

I reconnected with some of my pre-injury friends from high school during my 40s, some 27 years postinjury, when I arranged our high school reunion and via Facebook connections. We are all different people now, with life experience as our guide. It was a very scary time for all of us in 1987, but many of us have found our way back to friendship, which has been a healing process for me.

I was blessed, fortunate, lucky and any other similar word to have a mother who never stopped believing in me and went above and beyond to find all forms of treatment and support that would help lead me to the pathway of a rewarding and fulfilling life and career. I am also stubborn. Nothing came easy and life has been a rollercoaster, but what a journey!

Your journey may just be beginning, or like, me, it may be years since your brain injury. It is never too late to start healing your brain. It is never too late to want to improve your situation. You deserve the best!

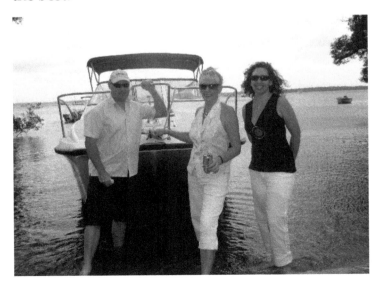

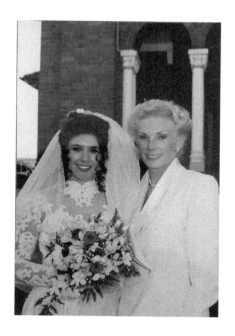

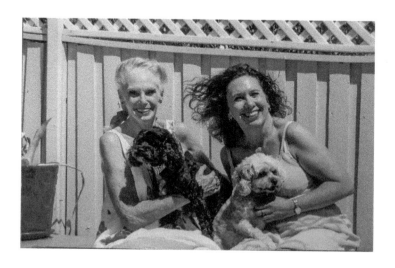

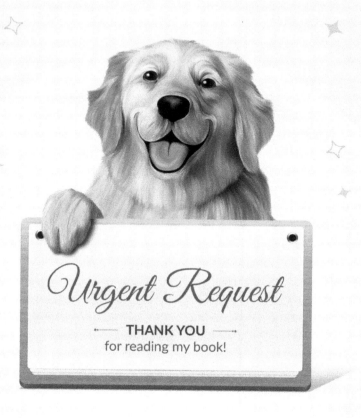

Urgent Request

—— **THANK YOU** ——

for reading my book!

I sincerely appreciate your feedback on my book, and I would love to hear what you have to say.

Please leave me a helpful review on Amazon letting me know what you thought of the book.

Thank you so much!

Nicole Yeates

Bibliography

Baycrest Centre for Geriatric Care. (2008). Injured Brains 'Work Harder' To Perform At Same Level As Healthy People. ScienceDaily. https://www.sciencedaily.com/releases/2008/09/080908185125.htm

Cheng, L., Cortese, D., Monti, M., Wang, F., Riganello, F., Arcuri, F., Di, H., and Schnakers, C. (2018). Do Sensory Stimulation Programs Have an Impact on Consciousness Recovery? *Frontiers in Neurology*, Vol 9. https://www.ncbi.nlm.nih.gov/pmc/articles/PMC6176776/

Doidge, N. (2015). *The Brain's Way of Healing*

Fernandez, I. (2019). Think Like Thomas Edison: Top 30 Life Lessons from Thomas Edison. Amazon.

Hensch, D. (2016). Positively Resilient. Red Wheel Weiser. Kindle Edition.

Johansson, B. & Rönnbäck, L. (2014). Long-Lasting Mental Fatigue After Traumatic Brain Injury – A Major Problem Most Often Neglected. Diagnostic Criteria, Assessment, Relation to Emotional and Cognitive Problems, Cellular Background, and Aspects on Treatment. Traumatic Brain Injury. Farid Sadaka, IntechOpen, DOI: 10.5772/57311

Millican-Hartnoll, P. (2020). Life in Verse. Tablo Publishing. Kindle Edition.

Roig-Quilis, M. (2015). Oromotor Dysfunction in Neuromuscular Disorders: Evaluation and Treatment. *Neuromuscular Disorders in Infancy, Childhood, and Adolescence,* 2nd ed. Academic Press pg. 958–975.

https://www.sciencedirect.com/science/article/pii/B9780124170445000470

Salas, C. E. (2013). Emotion Regulation after Acquired Brain Injury. 10.13140/2.1.2308.6080, 24/04/2013

https://www.researchgate.net/publication/262563464_Emotion_Regulation_after_Acquired_Brain_Injury

Seligman, M. (2019). The Hope Circuit. Nicholas Brealey Publishing.